Do We Still
Need Doctors?

Do We Still Need Doctors?

John D. Lantos, M.D.

Routledge
New York & London

Published in 1997 by

Routledge
29 West 35th Street
New York, NY 10001

Published in Great Britain by

Routledge
11 New Fetter Lane
London EC4P 4EE

Portions of Chapter 2 were published in "The Hastings Center Report."
Portions of Chapter 3 were published in "The Cambridge Quarterly of Ethics."
Portions of Chapter 6 were published in "Perspectives in Biology and Medicine"
    and in "Second Opinion."
All have been significantly revised.

Library of Congress Cataloging-in-Publication Data

Lantos, John D.
    Do we still need doctors? / John D. Lantos.
        p.   cm.
    Includes bibliographical references and index.
    ISBN 0-415-91852-9
    1. Medicine—Philosophy. 2. Physician and patient. 3. Medical innovations.
Medical care—United States. 5. Medicine—Practice—United States.
I. Title.
R723.L35   1997
610'.1—dc21   97-11424
                                               CIP

This book is dedicated to my father
Raymond J. Lantos, M.D.

Contents

Acknowledgments   ix

1. Introduction   1

2. Postwar Optimism   9

3. Priscilla's Story   32

4. Why Should We Care about Other People's Children?   49

5. Medical Education and Medical Morality   65

6. Truths, Stories, Fictions, and Lies   82

7. On Mistakes and Truth Telling   116

8. The Perils of Progress   133

9. Do We Still Need Doctors?   157

   Notes   199

   Index   207

Acknowledgments

This book couldn't have come about without the help of many, many people. Ken Schuit, Bob Glew, and Frances Drew made my medical-student years special, and Richard Michaels helped me understand what had happened to Ken. Arnold Einhorn was the best pediatric residency director the world has ever known.

The whole community on Sassafras Ridge became a touchstone for this and many other journeys and inquiries.

I arrived at the University of Chicago when Mark Siegler was just starting the Center for Clinical Medical Ethics. Numerous conversations and collaborations there with Mark, Steve Miles, Carol Stocking, J. Hughes, Mary Mahowald, Greg Sachs, Lainie Ross and our ethics fellows over the years have helped shape my thinking on every issue in this book. Ann Dudley Goldblatt and I have been teaching a course on literature and medicine to college students for years. Our conversations with each other and with the students have been invaluable.

Bill Meadow has discussed, critiqued, and improved every idea in this book and offered steadfast support for this and all my endeavors. Arthur Kohrman has been a friend, colleague, mentor, and role model. Paula Jaudes has unstintingly supported every zany project and paper I've proposed. Larry Gartner recognized how important it was to incorporate medical ethics into pediatric research and practice. Christine Cassel helped me grow and develop in a hundred ways, and Arthur

Rubenstein and Herb Abelson are innovative department chairs at a time when it is much easier just to focus on the bottom line.

Lauren Lantos reviewed and copyedited an earlier draft of the manuscript and made numerous valuable suggestions; Carl Elliot, Lance Stell, and Lainie Ross offered valuable insights into the strengths and weaknesses of the project; and conversations with Joel Frader, Neil Ward, and the narrative group at University of Illinois all helped me sharpen the central ideas of the book. Preliminary versions of many of the chapters were presented at conferences, Grand Rounds, and classes over the last few years. I'm indebted to everyone who listened, asked questions, and helped me refine these ideas.

Hilde Nelson first suggested that I pull my thoughts together for this book, encouraged me to write it, and edited an early version of the manuscript with acuity and humor.

Hannah, Tess, and Emma put up with all sorts of nonsense from their dad as the book came together—the nights and early mornings at the word processor, the repeated trips to present papers that became chapters, the anger and despair when things weren't coming together.

Nancy offered more steadfast support than everyone else put together and, more importantly, continuous faith in me and in the importance of the project.

1

Introduction

Do we still need doctors? The question may seem disingenuous. "Of course," the answer might go; "the sick, like the poor, will always be with us. Who else would care for them?" But to answer a question with a question would only lead to more questions, some of which might have disturbing answers. Many other professionals can care for the sick. Doctors do many things other than caring for the sick. The purpose of this book is to think about roles and responsibilities within that ever-metastasizing enterprise that we call the health care system. Particularly, I want to think about what doctors do within that system, what doctors once did, what doctors ought to do, and where lines should or could be drawn to define these various domains.

To think about how we might conceptualize what does or does not make someone a doctor is to stumble into an interesting morass. We have to know not only what doctors do or don't do but also how well or poorly they do specific things compared to other professionals. We might ask whether one needs to be a doctor to deliver a baby, or to determine which types of lenses best correct myopic vision, or to counsel the emotionally distressed. Should only doctors perform physical examinations, or administer anesthesia, or determine whether a patient is ready to be discharged from the hospital? Should we leave it to doctors to determine whether another doctor was negligent in a particular situation? How do we define and measure quality in order to decide whether doctors do these tasks better or worse than other people? And how do we decide appropriate reimbursement for the completion of the tasks? All of them have been and may be performed by doctors, but they may also be and often are performed by others.

Once we begin to ask such questions, subsidiary questions immediately spring to mind. How should we train doctors? Is the current premedical curriculum, which was developed in the late nineteenth century and which requires courses in calculus and physics but not in economics, public policy, or psychology, still appropriate as both an intellectual prerequisite and a significant part of the selection process for admission to medical school? There have been some important changes in medicine and the delivery of health services since 1890. Are internships and residencies crucial to the training of competent physicians, or are they an institutionalized and sadistic form of slave labor designed primarily to balance the budgets of teaching hospitals? Is it more important for a doctor to develop long-term and trusting relationships with patients or to develop expertise in a narrow but crucial aspect of therapy? Are there many things that doctors now do that could be done more competently and less expensively by other professionals?

In the real world of health care delivery and in the metaworld of health policy analysis, such questions are being asked, answers are being proposed, and policies that incorporate those answers are being implemented every day. Questions are asked and answered both implicitly and explicitly. Nobody knows which answers will turn out to be *right*. More interesting, it is hard even to agree about what it means for an answer to be "right." The measure of "rightness" could be specific and measurable improvements in the health of the population, such as lower infant mortality or a higher rate of vaccination against influenza. The measure of "rightness" could be the profitability of corporations in a challenging and competitive medical marketplace. It might include the satisfaction of patients, or a moral conception of what the medical profession ought to be, or an idea of the meaning of health and disease. It could be any combination of these or other metrics. Each would lead us in a certain direction. Without some sense of which answer is correct and, thus, in which direction we want to go, it is hard to evaluate the far-reaching changes that we are seeing in the world of medicine, biology, and health care delivery.

Doctors sense that things are changing but can't quite understand whether they should support or oppose the changes. Many feel overwhelmed, powerless, betrayed, and angry. Part of the frustration arises because of the way that the changes are occurring. They don't seem to be the arbitrary results of whim or fashion, but they also don't seem to be the result of careful planning or accountable political processes. They seem directed and inexorable, but nobody seems responsible. They seem to have a momentum, and a morality, and perhaps even a mind of their own.

For some, the changes seem to reflect the healthy and long-overdue recognition that medicine, like other social endeavors, is governed by economic laws. There are many attempts to describe the transformation of health care using the language of business and industry—to talk of the corporatization[1] or monetarization[2] of health care. These analyses generally describe the changes we are seeing and argue either for or against them, but few attempt to explain them. Even though we have understood economics for centuries, we never before thought that it should be applied to medicine in the ways that we now do. Why now?

For others, the current changes reflect advances in clinical science and clinical epidemiology that allow us to measure what works or doesn't work in a way that we never could before. In this view, the current changes are part of a trend toward higher quality care, fewer unwarranted variations in care, or greater accountability of care. Each of these interpretations of the current changes is undoubtedly part of the puzzle, but all seem unsatisfying to anyone who is looking for someone to blame.

We like to look for villains. It might be the meddlesome government, or the selfish lawyers, or the malingering patients, or the greedy for-profit health care chains. In a sense, it doesn't seem to matter who it is, as long as it is somebody. But it might not be anybody. It may be that the changes have come about because of subtle but pervasive shifts in what we, as a society, mean by and expect of medicine and health care and the professionals who provide it. Perhaps we don't need many of the things that doctors used to do. If so, then today's changes may reflect something more profound than market consolidation or better health services research. They may reflect a new way of understanding illness and a new way of responding to it that is so profound and far-reaching that it is both immensely threatening and damnably difficult to grasp.

Clearly, such a shift has been taking place. Countless writers have noted that a fundamental change in doctoring began as biologic science advanced to the point where medical treatment began to work. Prior to the twentieth century, medicine was a form of healing that primarily involved and inevitably required a relationship between a healer and a patient. Such medicine was a spiritual discipline for healer and patient, both of whom needed to recognize and harness the implicit and inherent powers of biologic organisms to heal themselves. Both worked to direct those powers toward certain goals. The process of healing was slow and frightening. It took patience and faith.

With advances in biologic science, we have begun to scratch the surface of a whole new domain of medical knowledge. We have learned to effectuate cures in ways that do not involve belief or human relationships. This change began sometime in the early twentieth century and led to a fundamental reconception of the role of a doctor. To the extent that the science and technology of medicine begins to work, the traditional role of the doctor can and does change from healer or comforter or shaman to scientist or technician or health care provider. Put another way, all of the emotional or spiritual qualities of the doctor-patient relationship that once were the essence of healing are no longer always necessary for healing to take place. The new medicine can work on patients who don't know their doctors or don't like their doctors. It can work on patients who are unconscious. It can make people unconscious. It can change the way people think, or see, or feel emotions.

We are just at the beginning of this new age. We are just beginning to understand the extraordinary extent of our new powers. These new powers challenge us to reevaluate the importance of many facets of traditional doctor roles. Some that once seemed central may become peripheral; others, which we may not have thought of as proper doctor roles at all, may become more and more essential.

Occasionally, biologic medicine stumbles upon a new understanding so powerful that it changes the way we view ourselves and our lives. The

smallpox vaccine has eliminated smallpox, and a scourge that was once
an inherent and essential part of human existence is now history. Oral
contraceptive pills have profoundly and permanently changed the way we
think about human sexuality and procreation. Organ transplantation
changes the way we think about death, bodily integrity, and the interrela-
tionships between people. Anesthesia changes our ideas about
consciousness, memory, and pain. With new ontologic challenges, we
reshuffle roles and expectations. We will always need to deal with illness,
suffering, and death, but we need not deal with them in the same way forever.

An element in each of these discoveries and breakthroughs is that the
locus of healing shifts from the person of the healer to the knowledge or
technology itself. Both the healer and the patient become relatively less
important, and the treatment and the disease become more central. We
no longer need think so hard about what the individual doctor can do.
Instead, we begin to think about what the system or the health care team
can do. Thus, a transformation is currently under way by which doctors
are becoming integrated into large and complex teams of health care
professionals. In such teams, the doctor is one player among equals. The
team members include other doctors; nurses; respiratory, physical, and
occupational therapists; social workers; pharmacists; nutritionists; statisticians; economists; hospital administrators; and others. These teams
work together to provide high-quality care within a fixed budget to populations of patients.

When health care is provided by such teams, we might ask what the
doctor's role on the team ought to be. Should the doctor be one team
member among equals, the star, the coach, or the general manager? Do
such teams work best when directed by a doctor or when directed in
some other way? To imagine that health care teams should be directed
by a doctor is to imagine that the current transition is not such a big
transition after all. Instead, it is a continuation of a process that has been
under way in health care delivery for a century. Doctors don't work
alone; they depend on others to make the drugs and devices, to do the
lab tests, take the X-rays, and change the bedpans.

To imagine that health care teams should be directed by someone other than the doctor, however, is to imagine a world in which doctors no longer do one of the things that define the profession: they no longer give the orders. They are no longer in charge. They are no longer the locus of responsibility for decisions and outcomes. Instead, they constitute one specialized health-service-delivery profession, one with expertise in pharmacology or surgery or physiology, among many fields of specialization. Such a change would have profound implications for the meaning of the profession. It might have more profound implications for our understanding of health, disease, and healing, and for the politics, economics, and regulatory superstructure of health delivery systems. Some think that such arrangements strike at the core of the doctor-patient relationship and hence at the essence of what it means to practice a healing profession.

If we imagine such a world in which doctors are no longer in charge, we must also ask who the new leaders will be, and how we ought to think of their roles and responsibilities. If the physicians are beholden to the leaders of large health delivery organizations, or to health-services-research czars, or to the guidelines and dictates of the latest malpractice litigation, then the people who run the organizations, do the studies, or write the legal decisions will bear some of the moral responsibility that we now vest in physicians. To whom will they be accountable? And by what mechanisms?

Such a world without traditional doctors would not be a world without health care. Instead, it would be a world in which a certain set of roles and privileges that we have come to conceptualize as inherently linked to the figure of the doctor would be conceptualized differently or would be obliterated. Such a world could be preferable to the present world. Some evidence suggests that it would be a world in which health care might be better and more cost-effective. Autonomous doctors create problems. They practice in idiosyncratic, uncontrollable, and often irrational ways. They don't follow rules. They don't regulate themselves well. They act in self-serving ways. They don't respect the autonomy of competent patients, unless threatened by a lawsuit. They bristle about sensible administrative controls. They generate enormous costs, which society must bear, for projects that have dubious societal benefit. They have a medieval-guild mentality. Perhaps we would all be better off without them. Imagining such a world of health care without doctors should be no more of a challenge than imagining a world in which we have shoes but no cobblers, trains but no engineers, farms but no farmers, or drive-through banks with nothing but automatic teller machines. Something is lost but something is gained.

The groundwork for such a reconceptualization of the role of the doctor has been under construction for decades. Specialization and subspecialization within medicine were a part of the process. Doctors themselves acknowledged that they couldn't know everything, couldn't care for patients single-handedly, needed to work in teams. Multispeciality group practices diffused responsibility for patient care among many professionals, each of whom was a physician but many of whom were not the patient's doctor. The process continued with the development of a variety of ancillary health care professions, each of which can carry out some of the tasks that doctors used to carry out themselves. Nutritionists oversee diet; social workers counsel; nurse anesthetists give anesthesia; physical therapists, occupational therapists, respiratory therapists, hospital pharmacists, psychologists, and clinical nurse specialists all have specific and specialized roles that are essential to patient care. Each takes a piece of what doctors once did and makes it his or her own professional responsibility.

These changes in the way we deliver health care prefigured and gave impetus to the current reorganization of systems for health care delivery. Some still imagine the doctor as conductor of this complex orchestra. Others see doctors as merely playing some of the instruments.

At each step along this path, there have been trade-offs. At each step, some doctors perceived that their role was being diminished and they fought the administrative changes that institutionalized that diminishment. Critics of change fought, and lost, against third-party payment, group practices, and capitated payment systems. Many are now fighting, and losing, against managed care. There is a rhyme and a rhythm to these struggles, but it is faint and difficult to discern.

The rhyme has to do with the diminishing importance of an ongoing private relationship between an individual doctor and an individual patient. Such a relationship, when it exists, can be important to healing.

It requires a special human bond. As third parties get involved in payment and reviewing records, confidentiality diminishes and the sacred trust begins to crumble. As group practices treat doctors as interchangeable, the process continues. Practice guidelines impose a rationality on this space, and it further shrivels. The rhythm of the struggles is the rhythm of twentieth-century American life, the replacement of the individual with the committee, the mass media, the bureacracy. It is a world that is both more cut off from traditional certainties and more enmeshed in its own rigid political and sociological structures.

To ask whether we still need doctors is to ask how these developments change the way we should think about the proper response to illness and suffering, how we should train the people whom we empower to respond, and how we should shape the institutions that educate those people and deliver those services. Such big questions cannot be answered head on. My responses to them will be somewhat elliptical. I will tell stories of episodes in my life and the lives of people I know in which disease and medicine played a role, and try to extract from these tales some insights and understandings about the way we now think about health and healing and about disease, suffering, and dying.

2

Postwar Optimism

A central question for the new world of medicine is whether we want medicine to be a rational, scientific, and orderly process. The new medicine aspires to these qualities. The new doctor is armed with new wonder drugs, new wonder statistics, and wonderful new analyses of cost-effectiveness and of the proper processes of rational decision making. There is a wonderfully clean and sterile hum to the modern hospital. Even in the intensive care units, calm efficiency pervades. Specialized teams draw blood, adjust ventilators, discuss the withdrawal of life support, and harvest organs for transplantation. The patients are abstracted into lab values, digital readouts, radiographic images, or moral categories.

There is something eerie and problematic about this calm efficiency. There seems to be no room for wonder itself, or terror, or tragedy. Disease and medicine touch all of our lives in intimate, profound, and frightening ways. As patients, we cannot want and don't really accept the wonderful abstraction. We insist on some recognition of our messy, personal tragedies.

Some time ago, my wife's mother, Evelyn, was diagnosed with breast cancer. She'd been living alone since her husband died of emphysema a few years before. She had nursed him through the last years of his life. As his lung disease got worse, his life closed in around him. He quit farming, then he had difficulty walking up stairs, and finally he became oxygen-dependent and was tethered by a nasal cannula to an old green metal tank that the home-health-care agency picked up and delivered the way he used to deliver and pick up milk bottles. At one point, the claustrophobia and fear became too much and he walked out into the road in front of an oncoming truck. The suicide attempt failed. He was hospitalized for a psychiatric assessment and started on an antidepressant medication that improved his mood. He lived another year and a half, long enough to see our third child, his fifth grandchild. She still treasures the pictures of her as a baby in his arms, pictures she returns to now and again as she rehearses her genealogy. He eventually died at home in his bed, a nineteenth-century death made possible by twentieth-century therapeutics. He appreciated what medicine had done for him but never had much good to say about the doctors.

Evelyn underwent a course of chemotherapy and radiation. It was tough. She lost her hair, lost a lot of weight, and was tired all the time. One of her daughters, Bethann, had moved back to the farm and helped out with little stuff: grocery shopping, driving to church, taking the car to get the oil changed. When Evelyn finished her chemotherapy and was declared cured, we had a family reunion at Bethann's house to celebrate.

We loved to visit Bethann. She lived with her husband in a house that her grandparents had built, on a hill overlooking the farm that had been in the family for generations. She nurtured a huge perennial garden and dried the flowers in the attic to make wreaths and wall hangings. They kept sheep, honeybees, and chickens; heated their house with wood; canned tomatoes; lived simply. At night, we could see stars and listen to cicadas. On the south side of Chicago, where we live, we put our kids to bed each night to the sound of sirens and, occasionally, of distant gunfire. When the kids got to the farm, they became different, more relaxed and open.

Bethann prepared a wonderful picnic for the family reunion. About twenty-five uncles and cousins, nephews and nieces feasted on fresh-picked corn on the cob, fried chicken, enchiladas, salad right out of the garden. Earlier in the day, we had gone blueberry picking, and the pies were just coming out of the oven. The kids were playing tag, the dogs were begging for handouts, the sun was setting over the rolling hills of northeastern Pennsylvania. The August evening light was mystical, wistful, almost magical in a romantic-movie sort of way.

After supper, Bethann stood up, grabbed her chest, and collapsed. She was just thirty-nine years old.

Bethann had had cardiac arrhythmias for many years. Nobody knew why. The cardiologists who catheterized her heart and studied the intricate and imperfect electrical pathways of her cardiac nerves declared themselves baffled. Maybe it was congenital, they said, or maybe she'd had rheumatic fever as a child that had never been diagnosed. Growing up on a farm, her family had rarely gone to doctors. To keep her heart beating regularly, Bethann had to take three drugs daily, some quite new and almost experimental. The drugs had side effects that left her feeling tired. It was hard to tell which symptoms were from the disease, which from the treatment, and which from the uncertainty of not knowing how to tell disease from treatment.

Bethann's disease was a tricky one. As long as her heartbeat was regular, she was perfectly healthy. When it became erratic, she was at risk of sudden death. She was a walking time bomb, and nobody knew the length of the fuse. She had troubled relationships with her doctors. They didn't talk to her the way she wanted to be talked to. Her "case" was fascinating, and they had trouble seeing beyond it to the patient, who was even more fascinating, or to the person who didn't want to be thought of as a patient. The very human encounter between doctors who weren't sure about the diagnosis or treatment or prognosis and a young woman who was both perfectly healthy and terminally ill at the same time was strained and constrained. The uncertainty challenged the doctors' power, and Bethann became the personification of that challenge and their powerlessness.

My wife, Nancy, and I are both doctors. When Bethann collapsed, we ran to her. Her eyes were rolled back in her head. She was gasping. Her color was terrible: pale, bluish-gray. We felt for a pulse. Nothing. We looked at her, at each other. This is it. I told somebody to call 911. We were way out in the country. Miles from nowhere. Better start chest compressions. 1-2-3-4-5.

Nancy couldn't do mouth-to-mouth on her own sister. We switched. She did the chest compressions. I started mouth-to-mouth. I had never done CPR in the field before. In the hospital, CPR is, weirdly enough, a friendly, communal activity. When a "code" is called, the team comes running, just as teams do on TV. There is familiar equipment. People work together. Anesthesia intubates. Residents start intravenous lines. Nurses, poised by the well-stocked "crash cart," hand me syringes full of precisely measured amounts of the proper medications. Monitors beep. In the hospital, you never do mouth-to-mouth resuscitation. Respiratory therapy has the ambubag. So I had never actually done it except on the plastic "Resusci-annie" dolls in CPR class. It was a little like that. Head tilt. Watch the chest. Puff. Count it out. 1-2-3-4-5. Breathe. 1-2-3-4-5.

In fact, it was nothing at all like CPR class or anything else. It was a gruesome nightmare. The sun was going down. We could hardly see what we were doing. Mosquitoes were buzzing by my ears. Kids were screaming and crying, but I heard them only like a distant soundtrack. I cut my lip pressing it against her teeth. My blood began to drip onto her lips and chin. With one part of my mind, I kept listening for a siren. With another part of my mind, I wasn't hearing or listening for anything, I was simply going through the motions of a routine that was as strange and mysterious as any prayer ritual, a set of motions and actions that I had learned to do in school and now could do well, even though I didn't quite know why I was doing them. This wasn't Bethann on the ground, this wasn't what it seemed, it was CPR class, it was a movie, it was going to have a happy ending.

Cardiopulmonary resuscitation has a central place in the imagery of modern medicine. Many books by doctors about doctoring, such as Melvin Konner's account of his third year of medical school,[3] Samuel Shem's bitter satire about residency,[4] David Hilfiker's cri de couer about rural family practice,[5] or Abraham Verghese's wistful tale of caring for AIDS patients in a small town,[6] start with a resuscitation scene. Placed at the introduction to so many reminiscences, this moment of dramatic crisis is presented as the defining moment in the life of a doctor, a moment when there is "nothing between life and death but my . . . hands, squeezing death out of the chest at seventy beats per minute."[7]

I remember two such moments from my own training. One was the first time a patient of mine had a first cardiac arrest. I was a third-year student doing a medicine clerkship. The third year of medical school is the first year when students get out of the classroom and begin the long apprenticeship that continues through residency. As a third-year student, I had my own patients for the first time. I interviewed them, examined them, tried to figure out what was wrong with them. Then I would tell the intern, who would tell the resident, who would tell the fellow and the attending physician. Although carefully insulated, I felt for the first time the awesome responsibility of diagnosis and treatment. I didn't want to make a mistake.

One of my patients was Mr. Gianonni, a garrulous seventy-six-year-old Italian construction worker. He'd been admitted a week before with a heart attack, had spent five days in the coronary care unit, and had been transferred to the floor. Like a good third-year medical student, I had spent hours taking his history. He loved to talk, so I got to know him pretty well. He talked of his childhood in Italy, coming to America, his marriage, his children, his work. He was charming, funny, and a little frightened. He seemed to have a lot of life left in him.

That night he had a cardiac arrest. I ran to his bedside and was one of the first to arrive. He lay on the bed, unconscious, gasping, and gray. I started doing chest compressions and kept them up throughout the whole code—the intubation, the lines, the cardioversion—although I was becoming more and more exhausted. As it became clear that he wouldn't make it, I got really mad at him, pounding on his chest harder and harder, and fighting back tears that came from missing him and fearing that I should have been able to save him. Inside, I was shouting, "Come back to life, you bastard." I felt that he had betrayed me, his vibrancy earlier in the day a sort of lie. The whole resuscitation was infused with frustrated anger, a feeling that Mr. Gianonni had somehow let us down.

Another time, as a resident, I was working in the neonatal intensive care unit. We had a 700-gram baby who had had four or five cardiac arrests. Every time we swung into action with the calm assurance of battle-hardened residents, and every time we managed to bring the baby back. We all knew the baby was going to die, but we felt powerful, snatching him time and again from the jaws of death. When we finished, we'd give each other high fives. Miller time.

Then, the attending physicians changed, and the new, older attending convinced the parents that it was time to let the baby go. An order was written to withhold resuscitation. A few hours later, the baby's heart slowed. We stood around the bed, waiting for the baby to die. To my surprise, he didn't. Instead, after about five minutes, his heart rate improved. Spontaneously. Just the way it did when we resuscitated him. What the hell? Were we just kidding ourselves? Has anyone ever done a placebo-controlled trial of CPR?

CPR is big in the movies and on TV. In our freshman medical ethics class, we use a *Star Trek* episode in which Worf, a Klingon, suffers a severe back injury. Devastated by his crippling injury, he elects to undergo an experimental procedure—"gentropic replication" of his spinal cord and a spinal cord transplant—that has never been tried before (except on Androids). It doesn't work. Worf gradually slips away on the operating room table. The resuscitation is vigorous, filled with the desperate urgency that seems to symbolize all that is best about modern medicine. The doctor is decisive, angrily committed to life, personally affronted when Worf dies. Or apparently dies. Just as our preemie got better with or without resuscitation, Worf got better in spite of resuscitation. Klingons, it turns out, have a backup central nervous system that kicks in if the primary one fails. It is never explained how or why the doctors didn't know that, and, as you watch, it doesn't really seem to matter. There is a mode of television viewing in which we can hold emotional realism, science fiction fantasy, and incoherent plots in our heads all at the same time. In the movie *E.T.*, when CPR fails but the patient survives, revived not by the code team from Los Angeles County Hospital but by the steadfast love of his little buddy, we believe it. We want to believe it. We'll clap for poor little Tinker Bell.

The new spate of doctor television shows have lots of CPR, usually followed by a romantic interlude. Both are very photogenic, and both seem relevant to our lives in a realistic sort of way. They get the feel of a resuscitation down just right—the tension, the frenzy, the primitive physical exertion of chest compressions, the crisp barking of cryptic orders, "Epi, stat, start a line, hang some dopamine, clamp that pumper!"

One aspect of these portrayals is not realistic. On television, most people survive, even if the odds are against them, just like Worf and E.T. The scriptwriters tease us with the possibility of failure, and then gratify us with a Disney ending. Our favorite characters live forever. In real life, survival rates after CPR range from 5 to 30 percent. Many survivors have neurologic damage and long-term disability. On three of the most popular television shows, according to a recent study, survival rates for patients who received CPR were between 60 and 100 percent. None of the survivors had serious neurologic sequelae.[8]

Television offers a peculiar melange of images and information. It plays into our anxious curiosity about doctors and medicine, and offers what purports to be total immersion and veracity. The backdrops are realistic, the clothes are right, the medical scenarios are gritty and honest. But at a certain point, reality becomes too much, and, in subtle ways, we return to romance. We don't want to take our medical reality straight. In the part of our selves that finds movies more interesting than medical journal articles, we don't believe that medicine is an orderly, straightforward endeavor. We believe in miracles and wonders.

Cardiopulmonary resuscitation has become the focus of one of the most hard-fought debates in contemporary medical ethics. The debate is about whether a doctor must provide treatments such as CPR even in situations in which the doctor thinks that it would be completely ineffective. The debate began with a focus on CPR for terminally ill cancer patients[9] and extremely premature newborns.[10] It has since spawned a voluminous literature and a number of legal cases but remains as contentious and unresolvable as it was when it began.

The inchoate and inconclusive debate about whether and how to designate certain treatments as "futile" and the inability of television or the movies to portray dismal reality accurately both take place at the murky interface between hope, trust, rationality, and medicine. Doctors used to offer hope even when there was none. Today, instead, we try to offer truth, which is better in some ways but less sustaining in others. Case-by-case debates about whether a particular treatment ought to be deemed futile for a particular patient are small examples of a much larger societal debate about the way we allocate resources for health care. We need to decide whether we want resources allocated in a way that does the most good or whether we want to incorporate other symbolic values. Is it ever OK to provide CPR even though it won't work as a way of declaring our loyalty and commitment to life, as a way of acting out our anger toward death or simply as an end-of-life ritual? Is it OK to have a health care system that doesn't efficiently produce the most health per dollar expended if it allows the protection of other important values? Our views about such matters seem to be shaped more by television's fictions than by medicine's realities.

The recent explicit debate over health care reform was, in many ways, an attempt to address these issues forthrightly. Our national failure to come to closure on that debate represents a flight from reality that is analogous to our willingness to believe the survival rates for CPR on television.

Clinton, Health Reform, and Postwar Politics

I had a unique view of the Clinton health reform process. In the spring of 1993, I was invited, under the false pretenses that my expenses would be paid, to participate in the work of President Clinton's Health Reform Task Force. (By the time I called the travel agency in Little Rock for subsidized plane tickets, it was too late.) I was a member of the Working Group on Ethics, one of thirty-five working groups assigned to analyze various aspects of the current health system and to propose changes that might be incorporated into the bill the president was preparing to send to Congress. We worked for months, putting in long and exhilarating hours trying to solve a puzzle that seemed to be a vast and amorphous Rubik's Cube. Every piece of the health care puzzle was connected to every other piece. Fix Medicaid, or Medicare, or Workman's Compensation, and you'd screw up the financing of academic medical centers, or state mental health care systems, or the private health insurance industry. Health care was a trillion-dollar-per-year enterprise, one-seventh of the U.S. economy, and had entrenched interests, subcultures, and lobbyists all sharpening their knives. We were at the eye of a storm so large and malevolent that nobody had predicted its fury. We worked peacefully in the deceptively quiet hallways and conference rooms of one of Washington's more baroque buildings.

The working groups were dismissed in the late spring of 1993. The president and first lady invited us all to a little reception on the south lawn of the White House. The reception was called for six o'clock, but we were told to arrive at five to get through security. Seven hundred people inched their way through metal detectors and strolled toward the Rose Garden.

We were used to metal detectors. The task force meetings had been in the Old Executive Office Building. Every morning, we would dutifully send our laptops through the metal detectors, then walk through our selves. We needed to bring our own laptops because there was no office support for the health reform working groups. Instead, we typed our memos wherever we could find a place to sit, and scurried around from the National Security Office to the Office of the Special Assistant to the President, looking for an unused printer. If only we could find a printer, we thought, we could transform the health care system.

The process was as inspired and as chaotic as its brilliant and moody insomniac guru, Ira Magaziner. He had a set of procedures that he imagined would allow all the different working groups to work simultaneously on different projects but that would create harmony, not dissonance. Each group was given weekly assignments, and at the end of each week we would meet in the Indian Treaty Room on the fourth floor. We didn't realize how prescient that choice of rooms was. At the first weekly meeting, the Work Group on Ethics had identified what we thought would be the major ethical challenges faced by any health reform plan. We suggested that the issue of rationing be formally addressed. Mr. Magaziner looked shocked. "There will be no rationing under the president's plan," he calmly informed us. The process went downhill from there.

The day of the closing reception was a lovely spring day. A military band on the White House balcony was playing jazz. Waiters, all of whom looked a little like Steven Seagal, were serving lemonade. There were no chips or crackers. No wine. The first couple arrived around 7:15.

Hillary thanked us all for our hard work: "Many of your spouses called the White House switchboard at ten, eleven, or twelve o'clock at night to ask if you were still working. I assured them that you were. I hope you were." At that time, closer to the 1992 campaign, innuendos about people lying to their spouses seemed bold. Hillary was in control.

Bill told us that the work of the task force was just the beginning, that if we could pass a health reform law, we could usher in a new era of social justice. The Clintons referred to each other as "the President" and "the First Lady." I wondered if their marriage was as devoid of intimacy as some reports describe it, whether they had this in common with the Roosevelts. And I wondered why we're so concerned about the sex lives of Democrats but imagine that Republicans don't have sex lives at all.

They told us as we were leaving that we should each pick up a small token of their appreciation. At the exit gate more military waiters were passing out boxes of M&Ms embossed with the presidential seal. The whole experience seemed dreamlike. M&Ms? Social justice? We had worked for three months in the eye of a storm of controversy and had just gotten fired with a kind thank-you. I couldn't imagine where we were going, and tried to think about where we'd been.

My father had just retired after a lifetime in practice as a general internist in a small town in Pennsylvania. He was bitter about what was going on in health care, depressed about what he saw as the end of a way of practicing medicine in which his values could be honored. He was tentatively hopeful that we might change things for the better. I thought about the changes he had seen.

Fifty years before our picnic at the White House, he was in the 29th Infantry Division of the U.S. Army, preparing for the Normandy invasion. He was an unlikely soldier. A basketball star in high school, he went off to a year of college in Ann Arbor and then, in 1943, he was drafted. He was nineteen. It seemed that if I could understand the story of how the war had led him to medicine, and to a particular type of postwar medicine, I might come closer to understanding the story of health care in our country.

The army tried to tell a simple morality tale. If you prepare well, you'll win. God is on our side. It started in boot camp. If you can run sixteen miles in hot summer weather with full pack, you'll win. Prepare! Individuals didn't matter, just groups. Stand in line to eat, to pee, to mail a letter, to buy a candy bar. Differences between individuals didn't matter. In the army, you worked with Poles, Hunkies, WASPs, and Creoles. Everybody but the blacks. He learned to shoot a gun. He learned to climb ropes to the tops of cliffs, to dig a foxhole, to stab the enemy with a bayonet. And all the while, it didn't seem real; it was just another basketball practice, another training drill, layups and bounce passes. It was a preseason scrimmage. If you did the drills right and got the skills down, you'd win. It was a matter of technique, of perseverance, of fairness.

Battle plans were drawn up. To Dad, they looked like basketball playbooks. The bombers go here. The paratroopers go there. Then the infantry will drive through here. It was like a give-and-go, a pick-and-roll. He knew how to listen to the coach, to follow the rules.

The night of the channel crossing, there was no moon, and the ships rolled on six-foot swells. The anxiety and seasickness took their toll. It was a queasy invasion force that hit the beaches at dawn. And when the door of the landing craft went down, the scene was nothing like the playbook, nothing like a basketball game. Things weren't where they were supposed to be. The path across the beach was being strafed by machine-gun fire. Everywhere soldiers were dead, or wounded, or cowering in shallow foxholes. Everywhere was the chaos of a riot, not the beauty of a play well executed.

Did anything that happened there help to make him a doctor? Perhaps it was the absolute helplessness and then the triumph, or the realization that technology alone got him off that beach and saved his life. Perhaps war and the death associated with it became a metaphor for disease and the death associated with it. The metaphor worked for Camus in *The Plague* and for Lyndon Johnson in the War on Poverty. Anything that causes disease and suffering is an enemy and can be defeated on the battlefield.

Fifteen years later, Dad would tell us stories at bedtime. My brother, Jeff, and I, bona fide baby boomers, shared a room in a new house in a new subdivision in the new suburb. During the day, we'd ride our bikes and play stepball or touch football. At night, we would lie in bed, under the unfinished eaves with rolls of insulation hanging down, on our knotty pine twin beds from Sears.

Most nights, we didn't get stories. Most nights he was too tired. He'd doze off on the sofa with a *New England Journal of Medicine* or *Annals of Internal Medicine* on his chest. That was when he still thought of himself as an elite clinician because he'd specialized in internal medicine, and board-certified internists were specialists compared to general practitioners. (Family practice hadn't yet been invented as a specialty.) He thought the journals were really written for him. Some nights, he'd get called out before bedtime. We never knew if he'd be there for breakfast in the morning. Other nights, he couldn't be bothered to tell stories, and we'd just get sent off to brush our teeth and go to sleep. But once in a while, who knows why, he would come up to see how we were doing, we would beg for a war story, and he would start to tell.

"We were supposed to take St. Lo on D plus two. But we couldn't get through the hedgerows. We didn't get there till the beginning of August, when Ike said to forget about casualties and get moving."

"Did you ever kill anyone?" I asked.

"No." Quickly. He didn't look at me and he didn't really look away either. His hands seemed to have a little tremor and his eyes went sort of blank. I wondered whether he was lying or whether he was remembering a time when he had killed a man, whether he remembered being scared. His memories never had any real emotion; they always seemed ironic, distant, absurd—memories of things that happened to someone else, a character in a movie, Forrest Gump. Maybe that's how he survived, by imagining that it was somebody else whose leg was nearly blown off because Ike got impatient. But watching him, I felt lonely and angry that he had gone to war in England and had never really come back. I wondered how many of them never really came back.

Then, "Nobody I saw, anyway. I was in a mortar company. We stayed behind the lines. We'd get eight or nine shells in the air before one landed. I have no idea where they landed."

They were parables, usually, about the stupidity of war. His own adventures were downplayed. He'd tell how he lost all his money playing poker on the ship home, how he didn't dig his foxhole, how his first wound was a bit of shrapnel to his earlobe. He didn't talk much about the next wound, the one that sent him home, but he'd show us the puckered divot in his hip and the lumpy calcifications around his elbow.

There was no time for questions. He didn't like questions. With him, the story was the story, and when it was over it was over.

Six weeks after landing with the second wave at Omaha Beach, he sustained a major shrapnel wound to the hip and elbow in heavy fighting near Brest. In one of the most efficient medical triage operations ever devised, he was flown back to Britain and operated on the next day. After three months in a rehab unit, he was sent home with a Purple Heart. One leg was a little shorter than the other, and he'd never play college basketball, but it could have been worse. Medicine was like war and war was like medicine, and both required discipline and preparation, and both required overwhelming technology. Both required intelligence and research. The side with the better radar, the biggest bombs, and the fastest planes would win.

He went back to Michigan on the GI Bill and then to medical school at Jefferson Medical College. It was the heyday of postwar optimism. Medicine was imbued with a transcendent sense of purpose. Just as we beat the Nazis, we would build hospitals in every town, triple the number of doctors. Heart disease and cancer would succumb to science, just as syphilis and tuberculosis had. Dad saw one of the first open-heart operations, the early experiments with renal dialysis. Penicillin became widely available and changed infectious diseases from killers to routine, treatable diseases. Laboratories started analyzing blood specimens for electrolytes, calcium, and phosphates. To the bewilderment of his father, who thought it time to get out and earn a living, Dad completed an internal medicine residency. Specialization was the thing to do.

Specialization and Managed Care

The need for specialization created a sociologic challenge for medicine. The exponential growth of knowledge made it increasingly necessary for doctors to rework the terms of their intracollegial collaborations. They needed to navigate the dangerous territorial shoals around the edges of their expertise. They needed to find a way to maintain authority and self-confidence while admitting that they had limitations and needed help, that others knew more than they did.

The first specialties—surgery, pediatrics, radiology, obstetrics—were defined by either a particular set of technical skills or a particular demographic category of patients, or both. But in the 1950s, specialists started carving out domains based on their knowledge of the diseases of a particular organ system. Such specialists would need to learn to collaborate in the care of a single patient, the cardiologist managing heart problems, the nephrologist managing kidney problems, and so on. For a while, it seemed like a solution had been found in the multispecialty group practice. Doctors wouldn't compete with one another. They'd work together, combining their areas of expertise.

In 1955, as the first board-certified internist in the booming coal and steel town of Johnstown, Pennsylvania, Dad set out to organize a multi-specialty group practice, then an innovative and slightly heretical form of practice. J. Dunbar Shields, an internist of the same generation, traveled a similar path. For Shields, group practice was a phenomenal experi-ence. He wrote, "My group practice is the thing I've done in medicine that I'm most proud of. . . . We talked about all the patients every day. We had a free interchange of ideas. What money we made was split in three equal parts. We never looked at the books. When you're practicing good medicine, you're learning medicine. Medicine was glorious fun."[11]

Group practices were pretty radical things. No longer could the patient turn to a single doctor with absolute trust and faith. Doctors called in consultants, patients had little choice about whom they might need to see, they'd tell their stories again and again, new doctors would order new tests, the price of care went up, continuity of care decreased. Anne Somers, a sociologist, describes the responses that group practices evoked from traditionalists: "The new methods of financing and organiz-ing medical services are often attacked as the causes of a significant deterioration in the relationship between doctor and patient, with a resultant decline in the quality of care. . . . Critics of the new financial and organizational trends contend that the patient's freedom is now threatened by the trend to large scale organization."[12] She wrote that in 1961. It could be a 1996 editorial about managed care.

Whenever an innovation in organization, financing, or structure comes along, doctors cry out that it will destroy the traditional doctor-patient relationship. And yet the past fifty years have seen nothing but innova-tion. Group practices, specialization, subspecialization, regionalization, the exponential growth in academic medicine have all chipped away at tradition. Today, according to critics, managed care is turning physicians into mere tradespeople, wage slaves in large and impersonal health factories. Soon, it seems, there will be no more doctors, just health care workers. (Ours is not the first profession to undergo such linguistic transformations. There are no longer any courtesans or prostitutes, just sex industry workers.)

The pundits are everywhere. Ezekiel Emanuel and Alan Brett, two physicians, fear that large managed care organizations will force patients to sever relationships with physicians, that patients will suspect their physicians of financial incentives to undertreat, and that patients will be victimized by plan failures.[13] Susan Wolf, a lawyer, notes that the new institutional structures will create conflicts between the doctor-patient relationship and physicians' loyalty to broader social goals, to organizational goals, and to their own personal goals.[14]

There is one problem with all of these critiques. They measure reform not against the present system but against a moral ideal. That ideal, however, never existed. There never really was a traditional doctor-patient relationship. It was always part nostalgia, part imagination. It is always so easy to imagine that times are bad now but that they were better once.

Anthropologists in the nineteenth century were fond of discovering undiscovered peoples in Samoa or Bali or Arizona and describing their "culture" at the point when it first was impacted by modernity. Anthropologists in the twentieth century have discovered that there is no such thing as an undiscovered people, that the pristine natives of Bali were as they were because of the influence of Muslim conquerors, Christian missionaries, Dutch colonizers, and Marxist revolutionaries.[15] Like the anthropologists, we must realize that the organization of health care delivery systems and the sociology of the medical profession always were and always will be compromises between moral values and political realities. There is nothing modern about modernity.

Dad's practice thrived in the fifties and sixties. He brought the technology of the tertiary-care center to Johnstown, introduced people to the diagnostic wonder of electrocardiograms, convinced the hospital board to build a new coronary-care unit, worked tirelessly to maintain a residency program in internal medicine. Like J. Dunbar Shields, he wanted the practice to grow. "We were going to have a bigger group," Shields writes, "so we could have more time off. We brought in a fourth man. His interest was cardiology" (p. 240). It was a time of hope. Like a lot of vets, Dad was entranced by John Kennedy's message of poetic optimism and mission. Kennedy made himself the candidate of the World War II foot soldier, the new generation. They would figure out new ways to do things, would not acknowledge that the old rules applied to them. They were the best and the brightest. For them, like for the NASA crew guiding Apollo 13, failure simply was not an option.

American politics ended for Dad with Kennedy's assassination. Along with a whole generation, he stopped asking what he could do for his country and began asking what was in it for him. Vietnam, the riots, and the assassinations of the 1960s just confirmed his view that hope had died in Dallas. His multispecialty group practice lasted until the 1970s, when the cardiologist got tired of subsidizing the cognitive specialists and set out to claim the $350,000 annual income that he'd come to believe was his due. The GI guy soon followed. A few years later, the practice was bought by the hospital, as part of its new Preferred Provider Organization (PPO).

A similar thing happened to other groups across the country. Again, Shields: "It wasn't long after [the cardiologist] came aboard that he said we were wasting too much time at the hospital. He felt the conferences were unnecessary. Then he said the business of splitting the money was not right because he was doing more procedures. He was making more money, so he wanted more money" (p. 240).

One of the more famous stories of such a dissolution is the story of the Marshfield Clinic, where, between 1954 and 1980, all physicians received the same income. According to Daniel McCarty and David Schiedermayer, who wrote a brief history of the Marshfield Clinic, the salary equalization plan "produced an esprit de corps, a feeling of cohesive unity, of mutual caring and cooperation, and it also encouraged innovations among the staff that set the tone for the future."[16] Like Dad's practice, Marshfield's experiment failed when it became impossible to recruit specialists because they could be earning far more money than generalists anywhere else. As doctors began learning how to play the Medicare reimbursement game, they began to develop practice styles that focused on the efficient production of the most lucrative aspects of their practice. Thus, it was doctors, responding to financial incentives, who began to fragment care and to charge separate fees for examining the patient, reading the radiograph, interpreting the electrocardiogram, the blood gas analysis, and the stress test. Each tiny element of care became a profit center, and each doctor who could monopolize a procedure became a player.

The nature of medicine changed. High salaries became the norm, and to generate the revenue, doctors needed to generate clinical volume. "Productivity figures have become the name of the game," reported one doctor at Marshfield. "In prior years, administrators were the servants but now they are in command. Reprimands or reductions in salary may follow failure to meet predetermined norms. Of necessity less time is spent with patients and relationships are less personal" (p. 264). The need for such administrative skills was not imposed upon unwilling doctors. It was the doctors themselves who created a crazily fragmented system, embodying the values that they created and promulgated, a system in which each specialty was out to game the system in whatever way it could. Managed care was not the cause of these changes. Physicians themselves brought them about. The need for someone to manage and control the doctors was the inevitable result.

The splintering of these multispecialty group practices may seem like a small problem, but it was a symptom of a much larger problem within medicine. Doctors were no longer all colleagues, all in it together. They no longer had a sense of shared goals or ideals or of professional solidarity. Instead of imagining together how the profession might respond to the scientific, political, moral, and economic challenges of the postwar era, physicians identified with a particular specialty. They imagined a profession that was infinitely divisible into smaller and smaller groups, into narrower and narrower subspecialties, and imagined that such division would be good for both doctors and patients. Doctors who specialized would make more money. They would also provide better care. Each specialty created its own professional society, and each society advocated for its members. Thus, doctors thought a lot about what was good for pediatricians, surgeons, or gastroenterologists, what was good for academic medical centers or rural family practice, but not about what all had in common.

One of the reasons that comprehensive national health reform seemed both necessary and possible in the 1990s was the demise of organized medicine as a political or moral force. Today, the once-powerful American Medical Association can speak only in the vaguest platitudes. Anything more would splinter its membership. Specific proposals for reform come instead from various subspecialty groups and generally reflect rather transparent attempts to shape policies that benefit that subspecialty. Though ultimately unsuccessful, the Clinton administration did learn that it could effortlessly play off primary care doctors against specialists, doctors in salaried positions against those who still work in fee-for-service arrangements, doctors who care for the young against doctors who care for the old.

The nonsystem that we have encourages physicians to look after their narrow interests. Self-interest is fashionable. Greed is good. We are all supposed to trust in the invisible hand of the market to organize these competing selfishnesses into lower prices, higher quality, and responsiveness to the preferences of consumers. Those who don't organize and lobby for their own interests get left behind. Faith in the market allows us to avoid asking questions about what a health care system should look like or the role that doctors ought to play in it.

In one sense, the answer to such questions may seem obvious. Cure illness, relieve suffering, decrease mortality, increase longevity. However, in another sense, that open-ended goal is precisely the problem. We do all those things, but the better we do them, the more we take them for granted and the less we appreciate them. And we can't decide how far to go. Is any expenditure, no matter how large, justifiable to relieve any amount of suffering, no matter how small? How should policies for health care compare with those for other endeavors that also relieve suffering and save lives, such as safer highways, more police, sex education, or cigarette taxes? In a sense, medicine has come to be perceived not as a solution to problems but as the problem that needs a solution. We begin to ask whether we can afford to waste so much on health care when we have so many real and pressing problems in other sectors. Should health expenditures always be granted the special priority they are given, and doctors the special authority to commandeer societal resources for whatever projects they deem worthwhile? In the postwar decades, the answer was unambiguously yes. Today, it is irresolvably ambiguous. We want to preserve some semblance of the doctors' special status and moral authority and hope that by doing so we can preserve some sense of what is special about medicine's particular ways of valuing and saving lives. But we also want to curtail the doctors' authority in so many ways that what we preserve is a relic, an icon.

Again, we return to a central question: Is the medical enterprise a rational, scientific, and orderly endeavor? In one sense, doctors want it to be. The authority of medicine is the authority of science, not of morality. If this is true, then we should be able to determine health needs, calculate costs, and measure the quality of sevices. We may never be able to specify precisely which tests should be done for which patients, but we should be able to measure and compare doctors, hospitals, and managed care organizations on many aspects of medical care. And we should be able to measure what doctors do and compare it with what nonphysicians do in similar circumstances—compare, say, optometrists to ophthalmologists, midwives to obstetricians, interactive computers to conversations with doctors. Doctors cannot oppose this without opposing rational measurement, accountability, and cost-effectiveness. And yet, such a project of rationalization is troubling. What if doctors don't do so well? What if we don't really need them after all? What if health improves and healing takes place without them? And what if something less tangible than a measurable improvement in survival rates seems to be lost?

A few years ago, Dad sold what was left of his practice to a growing managed care network. I imagine the buyers, in their pinstriped suits, sitting down in his office, opening their briefcases, and starting to talk about capitation payments, covered lives, and shared-risk arrangements. He must have had a sudden sense of childish bewilderment, as if he'd stumbled into the wrong classroom at school. I can see him nodding carefully, interrupting now and then to ask a question, excusing himself to go to the bathroom. It must have taken a long time to pee.

He's had a few health problems himself, but he doesn't have his own primary care doctor. When he has a problem, he chooses the best specialist, and when the problem is fixed, he never goes back. Perhaps that's how the informed patient of the future will behave.

When he went back to the office, the men were probably laughing. They had contracts on their closed briefcases that they expected him to sign. They were young, dark-haired, thin. They looked like they spent an hour every morning on their NordicTracks. He had nobody to call for advice, and didn't know how to ask. He was the person people asked for advice, not the one who needed it. He asked for a couple of days to think it over, but knew that he would sign. He was holding a worthless hand. They knew that he was bluffing. He was being offered fire-sale prices.

After retirement, Dad moved to Maine, where he spent his days drinking martinis by the lake, watching loons dive for perch, watching a family of ducklings grow up. He did a little *locum tenens* work as a utilization reviewer for a big PPO. I could imagine his glee as he asked specialists whether they really needed to hospitalize their patients or whether another endoscopy was really necessary. He seemed pretty happy.

He told me a joke recently about the director of a large HMO who died and went to heaven. Saint Peter asked him, "What did you do on earth?" "I was the director of a large managed care organization," he replied. "Hmmm, that's a tough one, wait here." Saint Peter went in, punched away at his computer for a while, and eventually returned, saying, "Good news. I got you three days."

The interesting thing about this joke is the unwitting compliment it pays to health care by likening it to heaven. It is as if we would all want to be in hospitals for eternity, and it's just the administrators who keep us out. But that vision is not of heaven but of hell. The better we get at keeping sicker and sicker people alive, so that everybody gets longer and longer stays in the ICU at greater and greater cost, the worse off everyone will be. The utopia of modern medicine is a curious one indeed; in it, the ultimate value of longevity and individual rights goes unquestioned. René Dubos noted that "all changes, even the most desirable, are always fraught with unpredictable consequences. The scientist must be beware of having to admit, like Captain Ahab in Melville's *Moby Dick*, 'All my means are sane. My motives and objects are mad.'"[17]

Bethann's resuscitation started with the best of motives but gradually became madness. We pumped and breathed away, the two doctors, providing what we optimistically think of as basic life support but which was really just a grisly sort of last rites. For a brief moment, I realized that all I was really doing was kissing Bethann good-bye, but then I heard the sirens and I blocked the thought from my mind. In CPR class, you learn to continue until help arrives or exhaustion ensues. The paramedics took over and continued the ritual all the way to the hospital.

After Bethann died, Nancy and I both tortured ourselves with questions. Did we do everything right? Might we have done better or was her resuscitation futile from the start? We both felt like shit. We had failed. But a funny thing happened. Everybody else told us how glad they were that we were there, and how comforting it was to know that Bethann had received CPR. They had the feeling that although she had died, she had somehow died properly. Our presence gave it a closure. We harbored doubts, but others were secure. We may have failed technically, but we had succeeded ritualistically.

B. Traven wrote a great novel called *The Bridge in the Jungle.*[18] In it, he describes the drowning death of a child in a small Mexican village as seen through the eyes of a white man. After the child's body is found and given to his mother, the man begins to feel a strange paranoia. "Any second, I expected to see all eyes fixed upon me as having been found guilty of magic or witchcraft and so responsible for the misfortune which had befallen that poor settlement of peaceful natives. Not so much to help but merely to keep my nerves from going to pieces, I assured myself that I was still alive and healthy by forcing myself to act" (pp. 120–21). The man goes to the child, who is already cold and stiff, and listens for a heartbeat, lifts the head, listens again, then silently turns away. "By my careful examination of the kid's heart, useless though it was, I had shown that I was willing to help. So I had been accepted as one of the mourners." Traven understood that as Westerners, as postmodernists, we can no longer authentically participate in the rituals of death except as experts, as outsiders, as mechanics, as physicians. Like the Westerner in Traven's novel, we have earned our right to join the mourners by sanctifying the death according to the traditions of modern medicine. Our work was meaningful to all who were there.

In his recent book about caring for AIDS patients, *My Own Country,* Abraham Verghese captures this sense of the comforts of medical ritual as he describes his examination of a dying patient:

I palpate Luther's neck, armpits, lymph nodes, I flash my penlight into his pupils, nose, mouth. I pull out my stethoscope and listen over his neck, heart, chest, belly, femoral arteries. I unsheathe my tendon hammer and tap his biceps, then his triceps. I percuss his chest. My tools—the hammer, the flashlight, the stethoscope—are scattered on his bed. As I pick them up, one by one, I realize that all I had to offer Luther was the ritual of examination, this dance of a Western shaman. Now the dance is over, and the beeps and blips of the monitors register again, as does the bored voice of an operator on the overhead speaker summoning someone stat.[19]

Whatever we were doing as we attended to Bethann, whatever Verghese was doing for himself or for Luther, whatever doctors do when medicine no longer "works," it doesn't seem to be rational or scientific or orderly. Bethann may have been better off dying in peace, and Luther's outcome was certainly not measurably improved by Verghese's careful physical examination. And yet, on another level, the operator's boredom about an impending emergency suggests a different and more appropriate ordering. The life-saving crisis moves to the background and the timeless rituals of caring and compassion move to the fore. We begin to focus less on the future and more on the present, less on outcomes and more on process.

John Berger writes about the difficulty of assessing the value of the work of an ordinary doctor. "What is the social value of a pain eased?" he asks. "What is the value of a life saved? How does the cure of a serious illness compare in value with one of the better poems of a minor poet? How does making a correct but extremely difficult diagnosis compare with painting a great canvas? In our society we do not know how to acknowledge, to measure the contribution of an ordinary working doctor."[20]

In the end, there is something ritualistic or symbolic about all that we do in medicine. Millions of children worldwide die of easily preventable measles or easily treatable diarrhea every year, thousands of American children have toxic levels of lead in their bloodstream from substandard housing, and we spend billions of dollars trying to save 600-gram preemies, to separate conjoined twins, to transplant livers. Whether what we do works or not seems like an almost meaningless question.

CPR will only rarely bring a dying patient back to life. But it will always be a desperate dance, a howl of pain, a brutal ritual of torture with elements of human sacrifice. We don't hurl people onto funeral pyres, but we mark their deaths by jolting their bodies with electric current, or sometimes by tearing open their chests. CPR will always be used profligately in cases where it is unlikely to be beneficial because we have so little else to offer and because, as drama and ritual, it works. We can't see through it. Until we come up with alternative rituals, other ways of dramatically affirming and valuing the lives of persons who are sick and dying, other frameworks for understanding and responding to illness and suffering, we will need these rituals badly. And as long as we do, efforts to rationalize health care, to make it efficient, to computerize it, to make it scientific, will miss the point.

Changes in the health care system may solve some problems, but they will exacerbate others. Disease and medicine touch all of our lives in intimate, profound, and frightening ways.

When I left the White House reception, I headed straight for the Farragut North Metro stop. I had to get to the airport and back to real life. I had patients to see the next day in my clinic for children with chronic disease, my clinic for the incurables. At the top of the escalator, a beggar asked me for change. I reached in my pocket and found the M&Ms, and handed them to him. "Bill Clinton just gave me these," I said. "Hang onto them. They'll be valuable someday."

For a moment, our eyes met. His were filled with both anger and resignation. The hopes that I'd raised by reaching into my pocket had been dashed when I pulled out something other than money. But not dashed completely. What was I offering? Was I making fun of him? Along with the anger and the resignation, there was a flicker of hope. Improbably, he still wanted to connect. "Look, man," I said, "It's got the presidential seal on it." He looked at the box, at me, back at the box. I tossed it to him. He mumbled, "Thanks, man." I stepped on the escalator and slowly descended.

3

Priscilla's Story

I like to go to Priscilla's room late at night. It is in a new wing of our hospital that was built for children who are dependent on mechanical ventilation. They are, in theory, preparing to go home on their ventilators, so the new wing was designed to look more "homey"—the furniture is made of wood, the wallpaper is more colorful.

Priscilla usually lies on her bed, looking up at her mobiles, and the monochromatic melodies from her music box harmonize with the beeping of her monitor and the low-pitched whoosh of her ventilator. I talk to her, tell her about my day. She is just a year old, but she looks back at me with eyes as old as time. She rarely smiles, never cries. Or never cries out loud. She can't. She has a tube in her throat. She looks wise, oracular, a mythic creature, half baby, half machine. The light at night is dim, a few fluorescent bulbs behind Plexiglas. Their white light flattens everything out. Sometimes, I imagine that I'm on a spaceship, me and the last child alive on earth. We're light years from the solar system, off to start over somewhere. And the mission depends on my keeping Priscilla alive.

She's getting a little bigger than she was when I first met her, but she won't ever get very big. She has a rare dwarfing syndrome called campomelic dysplasia. I had never seen a case of campomelic dysplasia, so I looked it up. According to David Smith's *Recognizable Patterns of Human Malformation*, "The great majority of patients die in the neonatal period from respiratory insufficiency, and those surviving into early infancy have feeding problems, failure to thrive, and evidence of serious central nervous system deficiency, including apneic spells."[21] Interestingly, the 1982 edition of Smith's book suggests nontreatment of these babies. The 1988 edition is less directive, stating only that "the oldest survivors include a 7 month old, a 19 month old, and a 17 year old boy with an IQ of 45" (p. 143).

I did a computer search, which turned up a number of articles in genetics journals about the search for a gene that might be responsible for the syndrome. There were also a couple of articles by orthopedic surgeons who had operated on the limbs and spines of children with campomelic dysplasia to try to ameliorate some of the disability associated with the deformities.[22] Calls to colleagues revealed that some recommend long-term mechanical ventilation for such children but others do not. One told of one child with this syndrome who eventually got off the ventilator. It seemed likely that Priscilla would never be able to breathe on her own. She doesn't seem to care. Or doesn't know any better.

It is peaceful in her room. The nurses don't come in to check on her very often, at least while I'm there. I hear them at the nurses' station, laughing softly, joking with one another about problems with their supervisor, or about men, or about troubles with their kids. During breaks, they go out on the porch for a smoke. Once, after a bad day, I went out and smoked with them. They made fun of me for smoking. A doctor! They don't seem to notice that they're smoking, too. Or they understand that in some strange way I am supposed to really believe the stuff I talk about, whereas they just work there.

Priscilla was born after a seventeen-year-old single mother's normal pregnancy. She had some malformations, a cleft palate, low-set ears, a small rib cage, and had some respiratory distress that led to her being put on a ventilator. After her cleft palate was repaired, she got off the ventilator, but at four weeks of age, she had a respiratory arrest and an emergency tracheotomy and was put back on a ventilator. She couldn't get off. Over the next few months, she was very unstable. She tried to die a number of times. The doctors were of a mind to let her. They talked to Mom about do-not-resuscitate orders. She refused to consider any limitation of treatment.

I met Priscilla when she was six months old. She was transferred to the hospital where I work, a specialty hospital for kids with chronic disease. We see it all. Diabetes, sickle-cell, asthma, lupus, short-gut, renal failure, cerebral palsy. We have a specialized unit for children who are ventilator-dependent. For them to get in, the parents have to agree to learn how to care for the children at home. At the time of Priscilla's transfer, her mother said she wanted to take Priscilla home and agreed to learn how to care for her. However, our program, like others, requires not one but two trained caregivers in the home. Priscilla's grandmother, with whom the mother lived, was to have been the second caregiver, but she and her daughter were not getting along, and shortly after Priscilla came to our hospital, her mom moved out of the house. The best-laid plans.

Priscilla developed seizures, which were eventually controlled with three different medications. She received occupational, physical, and speech therapy services. At fourteen months of age, she could do some of the things that a normal three-month-old could do. She could not sit but had good head control. She smiled responsively and reached for toys with both hands. She received all of her feedings through a gastrostomy tube, and she remained on 35 percent oxygen and fairly high ventilator settings.

She would stop breathing, periodically, in spite of the ventilator. Sometimes, she just needed a little extra oxygen. Occasionally, she required CPR. When her alarms went off, a "code" would be announced over the paging system, and nurses, respiratory therapists, pediatric residents, and I would all drop what we were doing, race to her room, and swing into the routine that we practiced every year on plastic dolls. We'd change her tracheotomy tube, insert large-bore needles into her shinbones, draw up and inject precise amounts of epinephrine, fluids, and bicarbonate. The resuscitations always made people feel heroic. The team was smooth, efficient. Each time Priscilla edged close to the brink of death, we'd haul her back.

After one such event, I brought up the issue of limiting treatment, and asked if everybody thought a DNR order was appropriate. People spoke rapidly, and with passion,

"I don't think I could sit and watch her turn blue without at least trying a little oxygen," a respiratory therapist said.

"I love that baby," a nurse said, looking at me somewhat fiercely. "When she's happy, sucking her thumb, and she looks at me with those big eyes, it's like she's calling out to me."

"I wouldn't want to just watch her die," another nurse said.

I asked whether her mother shouldn't be the one to make that decision, and whether we shouldn't be willing to help her with whatever decision she made. They paused, thought. Well, on the one hand, they thought it was certainly the mother's decision. On the other hand, Mom was just eighteen and didn't visit very often. They, the professionals, knew Priscilla much better than her mother did at this point, and Priscilla knew them better, too. They also knew her better than I did. I came on service for three months each year and made rounds for a couple hours every morning. They were at the bedside all day.

"Yeah, Mom should make the decision," the charge nurse said, frowning at me, "but *you* shouldn't tell her what to do."

I suddenly noticed that I was the only white male in the room.

"It's a personal decision," a respiratory therapist said. "We can't impose our views on her."

"But Mom's just a child," an older nurse said. "It's *her* mother who is really making the decisions. We have to make sure that Grandma really understands how bad the prognosis is."

"But Mom says she doesn't want us even talking to Grandma. We're supposed to start working with her auntie."

"If she was my baby, I'd take her home," the social worker said. "She might be the one that fools you, doc!"

She might be. After all, I think that Priscilla will die, but I can't say when. Because her ribcage will not grow, it is likely that, as she gets bigger and bigger, she will have increasing respiratory insufficiency and become harder and harder to ventilate. Unless we let her die during a respiratory arrest, she will likely die a long, slow death. But I'm not sure. New techniques for ventilation might come along. New operations may improve her ability to breathe. Geneticists are homing in on the gene that causes her disease—perhaps they'll discover a gene therapy. Maybe I'm being unduly pessimistic, blinded by a medical knowledge that doesn't allow me to see the everyday reality that the nurses are seeing, a happy little baby who happens to require a little technologic assistance.

"What if Priscilla's mother and I agreed to stop her ventilator?" I asked the nurses and therapists.

"No way, doc, that would be killing her. I couldn't do that. Couldn't even watch it."

"That's not what we're here for."

"If she wanted that, she should do it at home."

We went round and round, with arguments that were emotional, legal, moral, spiritual, and administrative. We were a group of doctors, nurses, and therapists, haltingly trying to tell a story about this baby's life and death that would make sense, that would make our lives as caregivers make sense, and that would end in something other than pathos and tragedy. But we couldn't seem to get the story right.

Her mother consistently missed appointments that were set up for her training. Her phone had been disconnected. On one visit, she gave a beeper number where she could be reached, but she did not always respond when paged. Once, when she did, I told her I needed to speak to her. We had a long talk. When I asked her what she understood about Priscilla's prognosis, she said, "Well, they been telling me since she was born that she was gonna die, but she ain't died yet." She didn't meet my eyes, stared defiantly out the window.

"As you know, we had to do CPR again the other night," I said, "One of these times, we might not be able to bring her back."

"Yeah, they tol' me that b'fore too, but seems like every time it happens, she just comes back stronger. Look at her."

We were sitting by Priscilla's crib. A mobile was spinning over her head. Priscilla was watching the little bears going round in circles to the music of a Brahms lullaby. A corrugated plastic tube connecting her to the ventilator gave her sixty breaths each minute of 35 percent oxygen. I watched the digital readouts of her heart rate and ventilatory rate, the reassuring sawtooth pattern of her EKG tracing on the amber oscilloscope screen. She was smiling, and seemed happy and carefree.

Outside, it was snowing. From the hospital window, I could see across the parking lot to the public school in our neighborhood. It is a dingy red-brick building that was built in 1916. The windows were covered with bars. The playground was covered with broken glass. There were no nets on the baskets. The mayor had just installed metal detectors at the doors to keep weapons out. Each class has thirty-five children.

Priscilla had been in the hospital now for all of her 440 days on earth. Her care had cost the state somewhere between half a million and a million dollars. Unlikely as it seemed, this 6-kilogram tyke was an engine of the economy. Reimbursement for her care alone paid the salaries of two nurses, a respiratory tech, a speech therapist, and a nutritionist. La Rabida Children's Hospital and Research Center is a private not-for-profit hospital on the shores of Lake Michigan. It is named after a monastery in Spain, a replica of which was built here during the Chicago Exposition of 1892 and later donated to the city. It has always been a site for programs serving the poor and neglected children of the city. At various times, it was a child welfare station, a dispensary for clean milk, a sanitarium, and a rheumatic fever hospital. It is now a specialty hospital for children with a variety of chronic diseases, today's waifs and outcasts. Our sixty-two-bed hospital is now the biggest employer in our community. I earn enough there to send my kids to private school, where there are nets on the baskets and the Internet is available on the computers in every classroom.

Although it is a private hospital, more than 90 percent of its inpatients rely on Medicaid to pay for their care. If their families aren't poor to start with, they quickly become poor under the burdens of caring for a chronically ill child. Many of our doctors were not born in the United States. Our nurses are mostly from working-class families in Chicago, some are white, some black, some Filipino, some Latin American. Many members of our board of directors live in the suburbs and run successful Chicago corporations. Our pediatric residents are from all over the world. La Rabida represents an amalgam of cultures and sits at the nerve center of a number of political and social controversies.

La Rabida's children are, in one sense, the dispossessed. We have kept some in the hospital for weeks while we waited for their families to get phone service or heat in their homes. Many doctors will not welcome such children into their practices because the demands are enormous, the outcomes often depressing, and the compensation low. A number of our children are in state custody because they have been abused, neglected, or abandoned.

In another sense, La Rabida's children are society's darlings, protected by a web of laws and regulations such as no children in the world have ever had before. They have a curiously indistinct and tentative right to medical treatment, never explicitly granted but implicitly spelled out in laws against neglect or discrimination against the disabled. This right creates an irrational patchwork of services, defined as much by the interests of the providers of those services and their lobbyists as by the needs of the children. Neither parents nor doctors may "neglect" such children, and the concept of neglect has been interpreted to preclude decisions to allow children to die of untreated cancer, prematurity, renal failure, or any other disease for which there is potentially beneficial treatment. Thus, children have become the objects of compelled medical interventions both inside the womb and immediately after birth.

Children have the right to an education, no matter how limited their intellectual capacity. We are prohibited by law from considering their disabilities when deciding whether to continue or discontinue treatment, although the distinction between their "disability" and their "disease" remains vague. They have been prohibited from working by child labor laws. Older children have been granted some rights to participate in medical decision making, even in decisions to forgo life-sustaining treatment. Each of these rights has been won through hard-fought political struggles. As a result, children have become symbols of political or religious positions, and decisions about children have become public, rather than private, in an unprecedented way.

At the same time, children have lost some of the privileges they once had. Although they go to school for longer and longer periods of time, the schools have been growing increasingly dangerous. Some children are shot by accident on school playgrounds. Many others witness and are traumatized by viewing acts of random violence. Many parents will not let their children go outside to play in the afternoon. Children seem to have lost the right to grow up in a safe environment. Instead, they suffer the emotional scars of children who have grown up in war zones.[23]

Death in childhood used to be common. Today, it is rare and excep-
tional. As death has become rarer, it has also taken on new public
significance. The death of a child used to be a private tragedy. Today, it
is a bureaucratic event, controlled by professionals and other strangers
and subject to the scrutiny of the media and the law.

Our changing views of both children and death create a turbulent
social and emotional situation where these two charged areas of interest
overlap. The deaths of children invoke all of the tensions inherent when
rapidly changing moral and cultural systems of thought and behavior
collide. Of course, there is a current set of moral and legal standards that
have evolved for dealing with such life-and-death medical decisions. By
these standards, treatment decisions should reflect an assessment of
what is best for the child. Considerations of what is good for the parents,
siblings, or society are forbidden. Generally, this means we err on the
side of life and do not consider costs. If either the doctors or the parents
want continued treatment, then treatment continues. Treatment can be
stopped only if there is consensus to stop among doctors and family
members. Even then, courts may step in and oppose such decisions.
Nurses are not formally involved in decision making, although they generally provide most of the hands-on care.

These paradigms for making decisions are well-intentioned but con-
ceptually shallow. Parents have rights, children have interests, doctors
have obligations. They reflect the expansive postwar economics of the
1950s, the rights-driven political philosophies of the 1960s, and the
technology-driven medical progress of the 1970s, all wrapped together
with the intense pragmatism of the hospital. We want to streamline decision making, to resolve ambiguity, to come up with testable and verifiable
solutions.

Increasingly, these legal and moral paradigms are coming under
unbearable tension. Parents are asked to make decisions that most cannot
conceptualize or deal with. Doctors and nurses are frustrated and angry
but tend to blame parents, payers, or one another for creating impossible
situations. Payers, public or private, continue to seek ways out from under
the burdens of paying for such care, and as they do, they increase the
pressure on doctors and hospitals. Interestingly, one response to the

breakdown in the current paradigms is to try to develop equally shallow new paradigms. Thus, we now talk about medical "futility" and imagine that policies defining futility will allow us to resolve successfully the dilemmas created by past legal, economic, or political policies. Or we seek new structures of health care administration, as if the problems we are facing are merely problems in organizational structure.

Children certainly have rights, and those rights deserve as much respect as anyone's, but they cannot be the same sort of rights as those of autonomous, independent adults. Children need to be cared for. The sicker they are, they more care they need. Such care is not a technical skill or something that a home-care agency or temporary foster parent can provide on a contractual basis. It is a moral commitment of the deepest and most profound sort, a psychological challenge that cannot be met without engaging forces that emanate from the core of our being. Children need parents, and parents cannot be conjured up by a court order.

Any policy solution that does not carefully and honestly assess the emotional and spiritual issues—as well as the legal, political, and philosophical issues—in difficult cases is doomed from the start. The feelings of the nurses and therapists that I encountered when talking about Priscilla's case reflect the complex and conflicted personal substrate upon which policies must be built. But current policies don't reflect those voices. Thus, theories and policies are developed that look good on paper but that break down when they confront the realities of people trying to care for one another. We play a shell game with responsibility, foisting it onto committees, courts, or corporate boards, but we don't talk about what it means for anyone, be they doctor, nurse, parent, judge, government bureaucrat, or insurance company CEO, to care for someone who is incurably sick, interminably dependent, or dying. We talk easily about heroic medical treatments but seldom recognize heroic emotional commitments. We seem a little confused about the proper boundary between the public and the private.

Kenzaburo Oe's *A Personal Matter* deals with this tension between public and private.[24] The novel follows a man, nicknamed Bird, as he deals with monumental decisions that must be made when his first son is born with a congenital brain anomaly. The story begins as Bird's wife is in labor. Bird is wandering aimlessly through town, worrying about the impending responsibilities of fatherhood, longing for his lost youth, and dreaming of running away to the wilds of Africa. The dangers of wild beasts seem small and finite compared to the infinite dangers of fatherhood, a frightening and ill-defined set of obligations.

The conflicts of ambivalent fatherhood are played out in a drama made more complex because medical decisions must be urgently made for Bird's malformed son. One group of doctors recommends that the baby be allowed to die. Another group recommends surgery, even though the prognosis after surgery is uncertain. Nobody can guarantee that the child won't be "a vegetable." Bird wonders about the moral status of such a baby, using imagery that evokes a hungry nestling:

> The death of a vegetable baby with only vegetable functions was not accompanied by suffering. Fine, but what did death mean to a baby like that? Or, for that matter, life? . . . What if there was a last judgment! Under what category of the Dead could you subpoena, prosecute, and sentence a baby with only vegetable functions who died no sooner than he was born? Only a few hours on this earth, spent in crying, tongue fluttering in his stretched, pearly-red mouth, wouldn't any judge consider that insufficient evidence? (pp. 30–31)

Bird initially decides against treatment, motivated mostly by his fears of what caring for the baby will mean for his own life. "I must forbid them to operate," Bird thinks, "otherwise the baby will march into my world like an occupying army." His mother-in-law and a former girlfriend to whom he confides his dilemma both support his decision. But he feels like a murderer. He realizes that he will never be able to tell his wife, that his marriage will end. Bird is caught in a dense web of conflicting loyalties.

The doctors are portrayed as judges or policemen. Each fact that they present demands a response. In each situation, there appears to be a right response, but it keeps changing. The decisions seem to be Bird's alone to make, but the doctors subtly limit the choices available to him, censure decisions they don't like, and try to bring him around to their views through intonations, raised eyebrows, pointed questions, or outright pleading. In his dreams, Bird is "subpoenaed by the tribunal beyond the darkness, and he is pondering a means of blinding them to his responsibility for the baby's death. Ultimately, he knows he will not be able to dupe the jurors, but he feels at the same time that he would like to make an appeal—those people in the hospital did it!" (p. 38).

The imagery of trials, tribunals, and last judgments that runs through the novel suggests that more is at stake than the life of a baby or Bird's marriage. Although intensely private, the decisions are also fraught with implications that extend beyond the personal. "With some personal experiences that lead you way into a cave all by yourself," Bird notes, "you must eventually come to a side tunnel or something that opens on a truth that concerns not just yourself but everyone" (p. 120). In the end, he changes his mind and takes the baby back for the operation. "All I want," he says, "is to stop being a man who continually runs away from responsibility" (p. 163).

In North American medical ethics, we insist upon a child-centered moral calculus in which parents are imagined to be rational actors, objectively digesting the facts given them by equally emotionless physicians and rationally choosing the option that is best for the child. Oe's work shows that this conception misses a crucial piece of the moral puzzle. There is a philosophic naivete about imagining that anyone facing parenthood can think in such a way, and a philosophic simplicity that borders on denial to believe it proper that they should. A more responsible approach to the care of children who are chronically ill and dying must acknowledge, as Oe does, the determinative role of emotions, the moral complexity of self-sacrifice, and the legitimate interests that must be weighed against the well-being of the child. One must at least acknowledge the importance of the burdens of caring for a child with a chronic illness and of the conflicting loyalties within families. Decisions about such children have interesting political and legal implications, but they can have moral significance only if we recognize and come to terms with the implications of offering parents the freedom to choose. The act of taking decisions away from parents, even when motivated by noble humanistic sentiments, is itself morally problematic.

I had the sense that Priscilla's mom would never take her home, that we were asking her to do more than she was capable of. Whatever the strange project was on which we were collaborating, it didn't have much to do with reuniting this family. But we couldn't quite figure out what it was about. The mother and I disagreed about the goals of treatment and even about the goals of talking. I wanted her to consider stopping treatment; she wanted me to leave her alone. I wanted to convey my concerns about Priscilla's prognosis; she wanted me to understand why she didn't trust doctors and didn't trust me. We were sparring about something, but it wasn't Priscilla. I realized that there was no reason on earth for her to consider a DNR order. To do so would be to admit her own genetic, emotional, and spiritual failure, to face some ultimate tribunal with no defense. She couldn't do much in this world, but she could advocate for the life of her little dwarf.

What if, I wondered, the next time Priscilla had a respiratory arrest, the residents walked instead of running, got to the bedside a little too late, took their time drawing up the medications, or failed to get an intravenous or interosseous line placed? Would this be dishonest? Or illegal? Such an approach is at least imagined frequently enough to have earned a name: "slow code." In a slow code, doctors and nurses go through the motions of cardiopulmonary resuscitation but do so in a way that attempts to minimize the chances that resuscitation will be successful. The approach seems to defy all moral notions of honesty, truth telling, and medical standards of care. Nobody knows how common it is.

Common or not, the slow code is probably a modern enactment of an ancient medical tradition by which doctors hasten death without revealing what they are doing. Many traditional medical practices, such as bloodletting or scarification, may have had this function. An illness is brought to a conclusion through ritual. There is willful and widespread belief that treatment is effective, without any attempt to examine the meaning of effective. It works in the context of the culture. Priscilla's mom and I may have wanted the same thing—for Priscilla to die a peaceful death—but I didn't want the legal liability that would come from taking responsibility and she didn't want the moral liability.

The present system is unjust in many ways. Resources are devoted to one patient that do little good, when they could go to many other patients and do more good. Resources are devoted to health care that might save more lives if they were spent on police protection or improve more lives if they were spent on education. We are drawn to the identifiable patient and make exorbitant expenditures to save individuals but cannot muster the political will to make investments that are statistically wiser but less emotionally compelling. We make analogies to the sailor lost at sea or the child who falls down a well, arguing that in such cases no expense should be spared. And yet, as medicine goes today, hundreds are lost at sea every day. We are all going to fall down wells. The moral imperative to drop everything for the symbolic commitment to save victims of freak accidents becomes harder and harder to justify.

Richard Powers recently wrote a novel about a children's hospital called *Operation Wandering Soul.*[25] In it, he tries to make sense of the world of children in the United States by imagining it through the eyes of a twelve-year-old immigrant from Southeast Asia who ends up in Los Angeles. She learns that the United States is a little strange, noticing that "the water coming out of the wall is good for you, but ponds and streams will kill you. The dead are not burned but buried in spacious, decorated plots, while the living set up house on a square meter of side-walk. Guns are legal but imported parrots are not" (p. 37). Her family is hunted by the immigration authorities until she is diagnosed with bone cancer. Then, suddenly, as a patient with a disease, she belongs in America in a way that she could not before.

Powers goes on to compare the glorious myths of modern pediatrics—we're conquering cancer, we're keeping babies alive who weigh no more than a loaf of bread—with other tales of childhood from other times and other places. He analyzes *Peter Pan* as a carefully sublimated tale of child abandonment and murder, in which the lost boys are abandoned children. He recalls the Children's Crusade, in which a hundred thousand children set off from a Europe in the throes of economic depression to reclaim the Holy Land. They never returned, but "travelers returning from the Middle East tell of light skinned Muslim slaves in Algeria and Alexandria who speak a strange pidgin of Arabic and Romance. This is the fabled end of that child cargo, traded on the international spot market, sold to the Saracens by creedless merchants, martyred to this round of teleology, an estimated hundred thousand innocents are lost, sold, killed, betrayed, evacuated from this world by faith" (p. 143).

And Powers examines the tale of the Pied Piper, which, as analogies go, perhaps most closely matches our current situation of crumbling infrastructure and atrophied political will. The rats of Hamelin destroy the infrastructure, he says, leading to a "negative balance of payments, debt servicing . . . graft, tax evasion . . . mushrooming social service costs" (p. 218). The Piper asks the city fathers to pay up in order to preserve life for future generations. They refuse, as we refuse to face the devastation of our cities, the generations of children growing up in American urban war zones where the war never ends. The Piper exacts a price by taking the children away. In each case, Powers notes how we transform tales of child abuse, neglect, or abandonment into tales in which children triumph. Kids don't die of neglect or starvation or wartime massacres; instead, they capture Jerusalem, disappear into the side of a mountain, go to Never-Never Land and never grow up. He suggests that in our modern version of such tales, victories against leukemia or prematurity or liver failure represent a desperate symbolic smokescreen to prevent us from looking at the realities we have created for our children and for children around the world.

Before we can choose among conceptions of justice, we need to see the little picture and the big picture, the economics and the emotions, the hospital and the neighborhood that it is in. We also may need to choose between abstract moral ideals and something that is both more human and more ambiguous. In our approach to death, the demand for moral clarity and explicitness may conflict with the way many people are capable of dealing with such issues.

Few debates have so energized bioethicists as the debate over legalization of euthanasia. Much seems to be at stake. Many proponents of legalized euthanasia believe that it should be permissible for people who are terminally ill and in intractable pain to choose how and when to end their lives. The examples often given are of patients dying of metastatic cancer whose brief remaining time on earth will be a time of unremitting pain. For such patients, however, it is clearly legal today to give steadily increasing doses of morphine until respiratory depression ensues. It is also legal to stipulate that the patient not be intubated or put on mechanical ventilation, so that when the morphine causes a respiratory arrest, the patient will be allowed to die. In such cases, the intravenous morphine is hastening death; everybody knows it, and most people, whether for or against "euthanasia," accept this as the morally appropriate course of action. There may be less at stake here than meets the eye.

To a certain extent, physician-assisted suicide is also legal. Physicians can certainly give patients prescriptions for doses of drugs that will be lethal. They can also instruct patients, either explicitly or implicitly (in the form of a warning that death will ensue if they take an overdose), as to how much of the drug has to be taken to bring about death. Patients are then free to take the drug, and if they die, the only question is whether to sign out the death as a suicide, an overdose, or something else. A physician acting in this way commits no crime. So some forms of euthanasia and physician-assisted suicide are clearly already legal, or at least are not clearly illegal.

Furthermore, most proponents of euthanasia continue to favor some restrictions on access to euthanasia, either procedural safeguards to assure that the patient who requests euthanasia is competent, or substantive limitations such as restriction of the option to patients who are "terminally ill and in intractable pain." Most proposals would also require physicians to certify that the patient's condition and decision meets the criteria. Few people advocate unrestricted access by any citizen to a quick and painless death. The issues in the debate, then, are mostly about where and how to draw lines, not about whether lines should be drawn.

By bringing the implicit and private decision-making process into the harsh light of explicit public decision making, proposals to legalize euthanasia or physician-assisted suicide may take the responsibility for judging the rightness or wrongness of particular end-of-life decisions away from physicians and their patients. An apparent increase in explicit freedom will be accompanied by an associated increase in oversight and regulation, and will lead to an implicit and concomitant decrease in trust. Like every other treatment decision, this one, too, will be evaluated by dispassionate bureaucrats who will be asked to ensure that some publicly agreed-upon criteria of moral appropriateness have been met.

But legal or not, the difficult issues will continue to be the same: understanding how people ought to live and ought to die; how they will understand and communicate their roles as caregivers and receivers of care, of being those with strength and power or of being those who are ill, blind, lame or, halt; and how they will make sense of the tragedies and enunciate a moral vision that will comfort those whom the tragedies afflict.

It is hard to locate the precise issues about which Priscilla's mother and I really disagreed. In my view, we would work as hard as we could to keep Priscilla alive unless we could explicitly decide together to let her die. By her mother's view, it seemed, Priscilla might live or she might die, but we shouldn't make a decision about it. A mother's role was to advocate for life and we offered her unlimited power to thus advocate. We had each other cornered in a relationship marred by totally incomparable notions of what it meant to care for a baby and be responsible.

In our passion for clarity, we seem to have developed a weird notion of critical illness: people must be classified as either living or dying. If they are dying, we know what to do. We go into a hospice mode and provide pain relief and palliative care. If they are living, we continue in a medical mode. But some people, like Priscilla, are, properly speaking, not dying, although they are at increased risk of death. They are not terminally ill, but they could die at any time. Their death, if it occurs, will never seem "natural." It will always seem to have resulted, one way or another, from a decision, a mistake, or a human action. In such cases, there is an inexorable need to assign responsibility, and an almost irresistible desire to try to avoid it. By such categories, we've created a moral gridlock.

There will always be questions of trust. Priscilla's mother didn't trust me, and I wasn't so sure about her. As a society, we used to trust doctors to exercise discretion in such cases. Today, we are suspicious of doctors and imagine, instead, that a more complex regulatory framework will give us greater protection from whatever it is that we fear. But the move from trust in people to trust in committees, institutions, laws, or regulations can never obviate the need for individual courage, honesty, and sensitivity, or the need for people who embody those virtues. The goal of medical ethics, it seems, should not be to develop rules that will minimize the need for individual virtues but to develop virtues that will minimize the need for rules. We don't need good systems, we need good people.

When I sit in Priscilla's room, I think about the meaning and value of her little life and of mine. She is more dependent on technology for survival than any human child has ever been. Looking at her, I realize that every breath I take and each step as I walk around her bed is a miracle. Yet, her care troubles me. What am I trying to prove? I perpetuate a system in which resources are devoted to one patient that do little good when they could go to many other patients and do more good.

But I like it in her room, late at night, when I could be almost anywhere else in the world, and I wonder why. Somehow, I am captivated by her eyes, which have never seen any world outside the hospital, by her bashful smile that seems tentative in the way that only a child whose caretaker changes every eight hours can be tentative, by the way her hands reach up to grasp a toy. She is the cripple who didn't make it into the side of the mountain, the lost girl who has fallen out of her perambulator. She is a sailor lost at sea, a child who has fallen down a well, cold and wet and scared and lonely. And so am I. We may not be able to save each other, but we can't just abandon each other.

4

Why Should We Care about Other People's Children?

When Iraq invaded Kuwait, a rumor began to circulate to the effect that Iraqi soldiers had gone to the Children's Hospital in Kuwait City and had taken premature babies out of their incubators and off their ventilators. This action was seen as particularly monstrous and served as fuel for the propaganda fire that eventually led to an ebullient national mood favoring the war against Iraq. Controlling the world's oil market was one thing, but any nation that would show such disregard for innocent babes deserved whatever evil fate President Bush could engineer for it. Such monsters deserved no pity.

It turned out the story was a lie. Nobody in Kuwait could be found, before or after the Iraqis left, to confirm it. It is true, however, that many children died as a result of the U.S. bombing of Baghdad, the invasion of Iraq, and the postwar embargo. A study in the *New England Journal of Medicine* that looked at infant mortality rates before and after the U.S. invasion showed that at least forty-six thousand deaths of children under the age of five could be directly attributed not to the war but to the postwar trade embargo.[26] Children could not get nutritional formula, or antibiotics, or hospital supplies. Clean water was hard to come by. Immunizations were scarce, leading to epidemics of diphtheria, measles, and other easily preventable childhood diseases. These were not the children of our political ally, however, and so their deaths were as politically irrelevant as most child deaths in the world.

Why do we care about other people's children? Apparently, one reason is that they serve our political and economic ends. That should come as a surprise to nobody, although it should embarrass us at least a little bit. We pride ourselves on recognizing the inherent and intrinsic moral value of children and other human beings. Citing Kant like a mantra, we insist that children have a right to be treated as ends in themselves and not solely as means to another's end. We agonize over the implications of this principle for policies about children's rights to consent to medical treatment or research, or to donate kidneys, or about parents' rights to allow their children to die. And yet, there is something disingenuous about our agony. Even a cursory examination of our actions suggests that our commitments to children are anything but morally pure.

We may have long ago banished child labor, but we happily buy many goods in our discount marts which come from countries whose labor markets we pretend not to know about. We may offer free schooling, but many schools have no books, overcrowded classrooms, rampant violence, and dropout rates that exceed the rates of high school graduation. We have child abuse laws, but most state child protection agencies are severely underfunded, and some are so inept that they operate under court supervision because they neglect the children entrusted to their care. In each of these areas, we make symbolic commitments to the idea that children have inalienable rights, but we don't put a whole lot of money where our morals are.

The problem is that children can rarely be ends in themselves. They have a unique moral status, based on their dependence and vulnerability, that leaves them always and inevitably passive. We make them do all sorts of things that they don't want to do, and tell ourselves that it is for their own good. Generally, of course, it is somebody else's conception of their own good. We decide how to raise our children by deciding what sort of values we wish to instill in them and what sort of people we want them to become. This, in turn, determines what sort of society we want ours to be. We care about children as a way of acting out a societal drama of moral values and inculcating those values into our children.

Even the adherence to a standard of considering their "best interest" turns out to be a peculiar way of endorsing a particular set of values that we hold dear, and accordingly a way to serve our interests as well. Each moral decision about and for a child thus represents a weighing of the degree to which we consider the child a means and the degree to which we consider the child an end. These are matters of degree, not of kind

It is hard to remember what it was like to be a child. No time of life is subject to as much psychic distortion as childhood. Freud knew it. The repressed-memory movement capitalizes on it. We reshape our memories of childhood into fictional idylls of carefree play and innocent beauty, even though anyone who spends time with children knows that child-hood is anything but carefree or innocent. It is a time of desperate struggle for love and affection, and of moral, psychic, and physical growth. It is a terrible and terrorizing time of bullies, random violence, abusive parents, and psychic terrors so horrible that they are trans-formed into the wolves and goblins, wicked witches and evil stepmothers of nursery rhymes.

One of the most bizarre but psychically understandable phenomena is the way we transform tales of child abuse and suffering into children's stories. "Ring around the Rosy" is a song about children dying of the plague. "Rock a Bye Baby" is a happy story of people watching passive-ly as a baby plunges to its death. If the best we can do to comfort our little ones at bedtime is to sing to them of abandonment in the treetops and a plunge to their deaths, imagine how horrible the thoughts that we are repressing must be!

In some ways, the best-interest standard is a similar sort of fairy tale, a transformation of our own needs and desires into an idyllic tale of self-less consideration for others. The 1996 political conventions were examples of this puerile hypocrisy. Both parties attempted to cloak themselves in mantles of "family values" and "child advocacy," but they were no more hypocritical than the viewers. By looking at a number of common pediatric moral conflicts, I will try to show how the best-interest standard comforts us with the belief that we selflessly care for our chil-dren, while, in actuality, other interests are served by the policies that follow.

Whose Interests?

In the previous chapter, I presented the story of Priscilla, a technology-dependent child with major congenital malformations. As her pediatrician, I care for her and try to keep her alive, often using brutal and painful interventions. Her life is frighteningly constricted, her future prospects bleak. Would she be better off dead? Am I serving her "best interest" by keeping her alive? I confess, I have no idea. I could argue strongly either way. I am clearly driven by her mother's opinions and make a procedural decision to defer to her mother's judgment about what is in her best interest, even though her mother clearly has interests of her own. The opinions, feelings, and values of the other health care workers also matter to me. And I consider my own interests, too, and those of my hospital. I "use" Priscilla as a good teaching case for medical students and residents, and I write and publish articles and books about her. Her continued presence in our hospital generates significant revenue. Her interests are intertwined with those of many other people.

Similar dilemmas arise not infrequently in neonatal intensive care. Premature babies or babies with congenital anomalies who survive as a result of intensive care may be left with severe neurodevelopmental problems. Imagine a male newborn who suffers brain damage and will be unable to ever sit, walk, talk, or care for himself. He may be blind and deaf, but he is clearly conscious, and continued treatment could keep him alive for years. His parents request that treatment be stopped. Should doctors honor such a request?

The best-interest standard would demand that we try to see things purely from the child's perspective. We should try to weigh, in our minds, whether continued existence would be a better way of respecting his rights than allowing him to die. It is important for us to believe that this reasoning process is the morally preferable way to make decisions for this baby because it validates a deeply held and core set of societal beliefs about individualism, about the proper relationship between children and parents, families and the state, morality and markets. We want to live in a certain type of society, one in which individuals are paramount and groups are prohibited from trampling on individual rights. We build such societal presumptions into every aspect of medical decision making, including situations like this one, where it is clear that the prescribed process is an act of wild imagination, not careful reasoning. Nobody, but nobody, can really know or fairly judge whether it is more in this child's interest to remain on the ventilator, to receive continued CPR with each episode of bradycardia, and to get the whole compendia of treatments that he is provided, or whether it would be more in his interest to be given high-quality palliative care and be allowed to die peacefully and painlessly. But everybody, no doubt, will have an opinion.

In practice, we resolve such cases through a set of procedural negotiations. Doctors and parents try to come to some consensus. Where they disagree, outside agencies such as ethics committees, child protection agencies, the courts, or legislatures may get involved. Federal guidelines that accompanied the 1984 Amendments to the Child Abuse and Treatment Act suggested that treatment should be obligatory if the infant is not comatose or the treatment neither "virtually futile" nor "inhumane."[27] This federal approach encodes a view that equates life with best interests. In this view, children are better off alive than dead unless they are comatose or the treatment itself is barbarous. No other considerations count. Many advocates for the disabled and many antiabortion groups agreed with this approach.[28]

Others have different opinions. In one study, 60 percent of pediatricians felt that such a rule did not reflect the best interests of children.[29] McCormick proposed that any decision process would need to walk the fine line between a medical vitalism that would preserve life at any cost and a medical pessimism that would kill when life seems burdensome, frustrating, or useless.[30] A group from Johns Hopkins University recently showed that babies born at between twenty-two and twenty-five weeks gestation had low survival rates and that 70 percent of survivors had neurologic abnormalities.[31] Although treatment for these babies is neither futile nor inhumane, the doctors suggested that it would be permissible to withhold treatment. They argue that when benefit to the child of continued treatment is statistically unlikely, then other interests may be appropriately considered.

William Silverman thinks that parents should be empowered to make such decisions, and that they should be entitled to consider their own welfare and that of other family members in deciding how to allocate their limited emotional and financial resources. "What happens," he asks, "when the dedicated actions of teams of neonatologists to rescue 'losers' in the game of reproductive roulette is not matched by an equal dedication on the part of parents or the state when the babies are sent home?"[32] Silverman argues that we have gone too far in emphasizing children's' rights over those of their parents.

It is not my purpose here to argue for or against any particular set of guidelines or regulations. I want only to point out that every group that has taken a position in these debates asserts that it is speaking for the "best interests" of the children involved, but each group also has its own interests. Pediatricians and neonatologists are no more selfless than parents, advocates for the disabled, legislators, or judges. Decisions about neonates take place against a complex web of social and political realignments, and influence social policy on matters as far-reaching as abortion, family policy, divorce laws, and medical education.

It is difficult to imagine a vantage point from which to evaluate objectively the interests of each group and the claims that they make. The attempt to achieve objectivity becomes an infinite regression of subjectivities. In the end, it seems that the only enduring conclusion is that we all care about children as a way of embodying a particular set of moral or political or economic beliefs. Children are always at least partly the means to an end in these debates, and their interests can be conceptualized only in the context of particular adult values or philosophies, or as instrumental in embodying certain ideas of a proper social order. This conclusion can be illustrated in other debates about the best interests of children in medical and social contexts. I will discuss three: the debate about growth hormone for short children; the debate about cochlear implants for deaf children; and the use of a best-interest standard in custody decisions.

Growth Hormone for Short Children

For the past ten years, a debate has been simmering regarding the proper indications for the use of human growth hormone (GH).[33] Should GH use be limited to children with GH deficiency,[34] to children with another medical condition associated with short stature (e.g., Turner syndrome or end-stage renal disease),[35] to children whose predicted adult height will be below a certain population percentile,[36] to children whose stature has been shown to be associated with psychological sequelae such as low self-esteem or poor school performance,[37] to any child who requests height-augmentation therapy, to any child whose parents request such therapy, or only to children whose parents can afford it? Arguments have been developed for and against most of these positions. As in other areas, arguments focus on opinions about whether treatment will or will not be in the child's best interest.

To the extent that these questions might be resolvable by using the concept of "best interest," three questions seem crucial. First, is being short harmful, and, if so, in what way and to what degree? Second, does GH therapy actually make people taller? If so, then does being made taller ameliorate the harms of shortness better than alternative approaches? Answers to these questions have been difficult to obtain.

Initial studies of the psychological sequelae of short stature suggested that short people had multiple psychological problems, but many of these studies were uncontrolled, retrospective, and rife with selection bias.[38] Larger, prospective, controlled studies have not confirmed the initial results. Instead, they show that any psychological syndromes associated with short stature are subtle and quite variable.[39] Furthermore, it is difficult to know how short is too short, or to know which short children will go on to have psychological problems.

It is also difficult to know whether short children will grow taller if given GH. Short-term, nonrandomized studies suggested that GH could increase the short-term growth velocity of children with normal endogenous GH levels without a concomitant increase in bone age.[40] Such studies suggest that final adult height will be augmented by GH therapy. A blind, placebo-controlled NIH study, which might resolve the question has been slowed by legal and political controversies. Studies in populations of children with Turner's syndrome show that final adult height can be increased,[41] and studies of children with other diseases or syndromes are under way.

No studies, to date, have examined the effect of GH treatment on the psychological conditions sometimes associated with short stature, or compared GH therapy to supportive psychological therapy. Furthermore, no studies have compared the psychological sequelae of short stature with other conditions known to affect adversely the psychological development of children, such as poor nutrition, single parents, exposure to community or domestic violence, or other problems. These comparisons would be useful in developing priorities for resource allocation.

With present data, it is difficult to say whether or how being short is detrimental to a child's interests or, if it is, how it compares with other problems that are also detrimental to a child's interests. Thus, some argue that treatment of children simply because they are short is inappropriate and that pediatricians, as guardians of children's interests, should not provide such treatment.[42] On the other hand, some pediatric endocrinologists treat such children and believe that treatment is psychologically beneficial.[43] Others suggest that decisions be deferred until more data from ongoing studies are available.[44]

Doing more studies is not an ethically neutral action. Studies, to date, have largely been sponsored by drug companies. In sponsoring studies, companies hope to develop new approved indications for their drug. Studies also support the careers of academic endocrinologists, who may become dependent upon grant support from drug companies. Such studies can be seen as ethically appropriate in that they protect children against fraudulent use of a therapy of unproven efficacy, or they can be seen as part of a larger scenario of self-interested behavior by drug companies and academic researchers in which children are simply a means to the end of generating profits for stockholders, favorable tenure decisions for professors, or the sort of data that might lead to approval of the use of GH for larger populations of children.

Further, decisions to do more research require decisions about what type of research to do. If height is good, is it an intrinsic good or an instrumental good? That is, are children better off taller because it allows them to do better in school, or are they better off taller because tallness is, in itself, a good thing? If tallness is instrumental, then GH must be compared with other interventions that might achieve the same end, such as, in the case of school performance, tutoring. But such comparison studies are not performed.

As in neonatal decisions, arguments of what is or is not in the interests of children become subsumed in arguments about resource-allocation priorities, parental rights, and the proper way to evaluate medical and psychological interventions. The interests of children are neither absolute nor unambiguous. They are always intertwined with the interests of others, and often must be weighed against those other interests.

Cochlear Implants

In 1990 the U.S. Food and Drug Administration (FDA) approved cochlear implants for children with profound hearing impairments. Since then, many physicians and parents of children who are deaf have opted to give implants to children. In spite of FDA approval and ongoing clinical experience, this therapy remains controversial.[45] In a 1991 position paper, the National Association for the Deaf (NAD) "deplored the decision of the FDA [to approve implants for children] which was unsound scientifically, procedurally, and ethically."[46] It insisted that implants should continue to be considered experimental because there were no data on the impact of implants on a child's social, intellectual, or emotional development. It pointed out that the FDA had received no input from scholars knowledgeable in the acquisition and use of manual communication in deaf children, and noted that many adults who are deaf decline to undergo cochlear implantation.

By taking this stand, the NAD declared, in essence, that it was in a better position than a child's parents or doctors to judge what is in the child's interests. How should such a claim be evaluated? In this situation, the issue is not whether the child will live or die, or be shorter or taller, but how the child will learn to communicate. Both the opponents and the proponents of cochlear implants agree that the goal of any intervention for a deaf child should be to develop the child's communicative ability. To determine whether cochlear implants are preferable to alternative approaches, we must evaluate the relative efficacy of each in maximizing communication skills in definable subpopulations of children.

The arguments put forward by the NAD focus on the child's interests. From the child's perspective, it argues, it seems preferable to postpone or avoid surgery if communicative competence using American Sign Language can be achieved noninvasively. Such an approach, however, demands much more of parents. Specifically, it demands that they learn a new language in order to communicate with their child.

Proponents of cochlear implants do not directly dispute these claims. Instead, they say, children who can only sign will be isolated from the mainstream of American society. Thus, they contend, an important factor in evaluating communicative competence is not just whether a child can communicate in any language but whether she or he can communicate in a spoken language. If, as it seems, children who learn ASL can communicate better with other people who know ASL than children who undergo cochlear implantation can communicate with other people who use spoken language, one must ask whether an important factor in evaluating communicative competence is the number of people with whom one can communicate. Thus, if a child with a cochlear implant can communicate only 10 percent as well as a child who learns to sign but can communicate with one thousand times as many people, he or she may be better off.

An objective judgment of the efficacy of cochlear implants would require studies that compare the psychosocial adjustment, educational function, and vocational outcome for two groups: (1) implanted children and (2) nonimplanted children who develop sign language in linguistically accessible educational environments. Such comparisons are difficult, because a medical procedure such as cochlear implantation commands societal resources in a way that educational interventions do not. Thus, it is generally easier for a child who has undergone cochlear implantation to get high-quality rehabilitative care than it is for a child who has not undergone implantation to get a schoolteacher who knows how to sign. Such implicit societal biases for or against different types of interventions make it difficult to evaluate objectively what is or is not in a deaf child's best interest.

Custody Decisions

The concept of considering a "child's best interest" was originally conceptualized by psychiatrists and social workers to guide custody decisions in divorce cases.[47] In that context, it functioned to discredit other approaches to custody decisions, such as rules giving automatic preference to either the father or the mother. As conceptualized by Goldstein and colleagues, the recommended mechanism for evaluating best interest in custody cases has been to determine which parental relationship is most psychologically beneficial for the child.[48] Courts rely on expert testimony by psychiatrists or psychologists to determine what is best for the child. Does it work?

Jon Elster has argued that the best-interest standard is usually indeterminate, often unjust, and operationally self-defeating.[49] It is indeterminate because we can never rationally consider every element that contributes to a child's upbringing. To do so, we would have to question whether it is more important to live in a safe neighborhood, to go to better schools, to have a relationship with an adult with whom one can discuss one's fears, to receive a comprehensive religious education, and to weigh each of these and many other factors. We would then need to calculate the measurable benefit and the likelihood of each outcome's being achieved, and calculate an overall best-interest score for each option.

Such a comprehensive process is, of course, never used. Instead, certain outcomes are implicitly elevated above others, based on the personal preferences of the empowered judge and an unverifiable assessment of the likelihood of achieving these outcomes. Often, professionals disagree about what is in the best interest of a child, and the judge must weigh the opinions of each side's partisan experts.

The best-interest standard is often unjust. Although children are citizens whose interests need to be considered and protected, parents have interests as well. Justice generally implies that a balance be struck among competing interests. The child's-best-interest standard proposes that no balancing is necessary. When originally proposed, this may have been justified as historically necessary to counteract a long legal tradition that treated children as property rather than as citizens.[50] However, a pure best-interest standard would lead to cases where great injustice would be done to a parent or to other siblings in order to justify a small benefit to a child. In such cases, justice may demand that although children's unique vulnerability demands that their interests be given special consideration and representation, those interests do not always and necessarily trump other interests.

In custody decisions, the best-interest standard can become operationally self-defeating. In most custody cases, a quick decision is best for children. However, because the best-interest standard favors the custodial parent, that parent has an incentive to delay the decision as long as possible. Furthermore, both parents have an incentive to denigrate the character of the other in order to show that placement would be detrimental to the child. However, such character denigration is itself detrimental to the child. Paradoxically, then, a thorough and comprehensive determination of what is in the child's best interest may itself be not be in the child's best interest.

The Political Economy of the Best-Interest Standard

I have tried to show that children's interests are neither easy to assess nor easy to protect. In most cases, controversies about children's interests reflect controversies about the interests of the involved adults and about the types of values those adults hold dear. Recognizing this connection does not, in itself, invalidate attempts to consider what is best for the child. Instead, it asks that such attempts consider how children's interests intertwine with adults' interests.

Once the connection between adult interests and the interests of children is recognized, it becomes apparent that even a policy of recognizing and emphasizing the child's best interests needs to be examined. Whose interests does it serve to choose this approach to resolving dilemmas about growth hormone or neonatal care or custody? Why do we choose to care for other people's children in this particular way?

The best-interest standard is theoretically interesting because it posits a child who is independent and rationally self-interested. Each child is assumed to want to consider only her or his own interests and not to consider the interests or values of her or his family or community. This is a somewhat peculiar construct because all of us, and especially children, live within dense social matrices. We all consider our own interests, of course, but our own interests are always intertwined, molded, and sometimes even subsumed into the interests of others. The best-interest standard rejects this approach. In doing so, it protects the vulnerable from exploitation. It also protects them from reality. The best-interest approach endorses and exemplifies a view of rational self-interest that is the basis of much political and economic theory and that has permeated bioethics in other ways. According to the dominant economic ideology of market capitalism, self-interested behavior is good, rational, and inevitable, and altruistic behavior is hypocritical or suspect. Benevolent behavior toward others is seen as paternalistic and demeaning. By this view, adults always and necessarily assess their own self-interest first in any situation, and this is what they *should* do.

We don't trust any system or institution that presumes to judge for others. Doctors are therefore not to act in a paternalistic manner, imposing their own views of what is good. Instead, they are to promote patient autonomy and self-determination. The good can be defined only procedurally. Whatever a competent person decides to do is good, and that competent person will generally act in a self-interested way. Somehow, through the magic of the marketplace, the sum total of millions of such self-interested decisions will result not only in functioning communities but also in the best possible communities, ones that most effectively balance competing interests. Of course, this will work only if there is initial equality in power and understanding between those engaged in the decisions.

Annette Baier noted,

> It is a typical feature of the dominant moral theories and traditions since Kant, or perhaps since Hobbes, that relationships between equals or those who are deemed equal in some important sense have been the relations that morality is primarily concerned to regulate. Relationships between those who are clearly unequal in power, such as parents and children, earlier and later generations in relation to one another, states and citizens, doctors and patients, the well and the ill, large states and small states, have had to be shunted to the bottom of the agenda and then dealt with by some sort of "promotion" of the weaker, so that an appearance of virtual equality is achieved. . . . Children are treated as adults-to-be, the ill and dying

treated as continuers of their earlier more potent selves, so that their
"rights" can be seen as the rights of equals.[51]

But of course, inequality in the world is not something that can be imagined or legislated away. Any moral theory that relies on the fictional
creation of an "appearance of virtual equality" will be a moral theory
appropriate only for virtual worlds. It wouldn't help me or her mother to
care for Priscilla.

The continued existence of children is an embarrassment to moral
theory. They demand compromises of us that we have difficulty account-
ing for. John Stuart Mill, an ardent defender of individual liberty from
state intervention, took pains to make a special case for parental responsibility for children. Thus, he thought that it was acceptable for states to
regulate marriage and childbearing in ways that would assure the well-
being of children. He wrote, "[T]he laws which, in many countries on the
Continent, forbid marriage unless the parties can show that they have
the means of supporting a family do not exceed the legitimate powers of
the State . . . they are not objectionable as violations of liberty."[52] This
was because "to bring a child into existence without a fair prospect of
being able, not only to provide food for its body but instruction and
training for its mind, is a moral crime, both against the unfortunate off-
spring and against society, and that if the parent does not fulfill this
obligation, the State ought to see it fulfilled, at the charge, as far as possible, of the parent."[53]

Children are physically dependent and morally primitive. They are
also the future of humanity. As a society or as parents, we justify all sorts
of coercive behavior toward children in the hope that they will turn into
the sorts of adults with whom we would like to live and who will carry on
our values. We do so because it is the only available means to reach a
desirable end.

But what is the end? What moral world are we raising children to participate in? We cannot decide which sorts of actions are appropriate or
inappropriate toward children unless we have a fairly thick and detailed
conception of the moral qualities that we think adults should have in
order to participate in that world. Do we want adults who tell the truth,

keep promises, trust one another? Do we want adults who take orders well, who make good soldiers? Do we want women and men to be more alike or more different from one another than they have been in the past? What views of parenthood might we impose? Should we exalt self-interested behavior or self-sacrifices for one another?

And we have to decide who we mean by "we." Whose voices should be heard in these decisions? How much diversity should we allow among families, and how much standardization might the government impose? Answers to concrete questions such as these are the groundwork of moral policies about children. Both the positive-rights-oriented political left and the negative-rights-oriented political right impose moral values on children.

There is a possibility, of course, that unbridled individualism might lead to bad outcomes. There may be situations in which we need some sort of protection from our own impulses. Such protection might include government programs that force us to put money away for our old age, systems to regulate stock trading or to prevent the marketing of unproven drugs. It might even include programs to care for those in society who cannot care for themselves.

Much current political debate focuses on whether these responsibilities should be assumed by the government or by the citzenry. This is a somewhat curious debate in a democracy, where the government is thought to represent the citizenry. Perhaps because of this, the arguments in favor of minimalist government are powerful. In the case of charity or welfare programs, the arguments go, people are either altruistic or they are not. If they are not, and the government is representative and democratic, then the government should not force the people to act altruistically, that is, to act in a way that they don't want to act. If the people are altruistic, then they should not need their government to make them act in a way that they want to act anyway. Either way, we are left with an argument for a minimalist government and a reliance on individuals. Unless, of course, the government can be greater than the sum of its voters, and society more than an aggregation of self-interested individuals.

I began by asking why we care for other people's children. Following this inquiry, it seems more interesting to ask why we care for particular children in the particular way that we do. In responding to the children involved in the Iraqi-Kuwaiti conflict, we showed extraordinary concern for some imaginary children and we were willing to participate in policies that led to the deaths of some very real children. We did so to demonstrate our wrath and our strength symbolically. Our willingness to implement policies that would cause children to suffer and die became a test of our moral purpose.

Everybody cares for other people's children because they care for the future of our society. Moral systems, like biologic systems, perpetuate themselves. Therefore, we must care for children in such a way as to instill in them a sense of our moral purpose. In this country, we deify the autonomy of the competent adult and assume that his or her uncoerced actions must represent the be-all and end-all of morality. We believe that such adults act primarily out of self-interest. Our peculiar sort of caring for children tries to reinforce our beliefs and to act them out in a way that will instill in each child the values that we believe he or she will need in order to participate in this society. We act as if children should be concerned solely with their own best interests. We treat them as selfish and self-interested creatures in order to teach them that it is proper to be selfish.

These core values of individualism and autonomy, which inform decisions about children, permeate every other aspect of bioethics. The powerlessness and vulnerability of patients in relationship to their doctors is as embarrassing as the powerlessness and vulnerability of children. We want to imagine that patients, no matter how ill, can participate in the process of self-interested contract making that is at the center of our moral vision of how people ought to interact. We have constructed a legal and ethical framework around our medical care system that mirrors and reinforces the social values we hold dear.

Instilling moral values in the next generation does not, of course, end with the parent-child relationship. Many other social systems embody and incorporate value decisions of this type. In the next chapter, I will consider some of the values implicit in our current system of medical education.

5

Medical Education
and Medical Morality

Dr. Ken Schuit was an enormously popular and accomplished medical school professor at the largest liver transplant center in the world. He died of liver failure. To the shock and surprise of his colleagues and friends, he refused to undergo a liver transplant. He knew he was going to die yet refused even to speak to the transplant surgeons. Instead, he slipped into hepatic coma and died after a brief illness. His refusal to undergo a liver transplant was something of a mystery. What was he trying to say?

Ken was a pediatric infectious disease specialist at the University of Pittsburgh when he developed fulminant hepatitic failure. He was also one of the most extraordinary teachers on the faculty and probably one of the best medical educators in the country. But this is a dubious distinction. Excellence in teaching is not something usually measured or rewarded in medical schools. Teaching is generally not counted as an important activity when it comes time for promotion or salary negotiations. We are suspicious of excellence in teaching because we can't measure quality, and things we can't measure just don't count for much. Teaching doesn't bring in grant money (unless one studies educational interventions); it doesn't lead to publications or generate clinical revenue. The only people who notice are the students. The only thing at stake is the future.

Medical students give awards for teaching. Ken won the teaching award from the students six times in his last ten years. He won a special chancellor's award for teaching the year before he died. Skill at teaching may be unmeasurable, but it is clearly recognizable. You know it when you see it. One would think that in a medical school, where the education of medical students is central to the mission of the institution, extraordinary teaching would be recognized and valued. But Ken had trouble getting promoted to the rank of full professor. (His promotion came through two weeks before he died.) He didn't get grants, didn't publish much. His wasn't the sort of career that any thriving academic medical center would want to encourage.

The students whose lives Ken had touched turned out in unprecedented numbers for his memorial service. A half an hour before the service began, there were no seats left in the chapel. People were afraid that the balcony would collapse. The line to get in stretched around the block, and many people waited outside during the entire service.

I met Ken when I was preparing to go to Nigeria after my second year of medical school. He had worked with another master teacher, Robert Glew, to set up an exchange program between the University of Pittsburgh and the University of Benin in Benin City, Nigeria.

As one of the first exchange students, I spent three months living in a poured-concrete dorm room and caring for babies with measles and malaria and neonatal tetanus. Nigeria was a happier place then. The nightmare of its Biafran civil war was seemingly over and Nigerians were attempting the transition from military dictatorship to American-style democracy. But even in 1979, when hopes seemed the highest, there was a sense among the people that tribal loyalties could never be erased. During my stay, the people of Benin celebrated the coronation of a new Oba, or chieftain. I was told to stay off the streets during the celebration, that the Benis were a primitive tribe, that strange things happened during the coronation of a new Oba.

I lost weight in Nigeria. I ate cassava root and yam, ground nuts and boiled eggs. Everything was drenched in red pepper sauce. I had fevers, night sweats, bloody stools, and heart palpitations. And I had adventures. I bargained in the market for tie-died cloth that I took to Yakubu, the

Supreme Tailor, to make into robes. Every afternoon, the billowing clouds would release a drenching shower that wouldn't even begin to cool things off. Like throwing water on the rocks of a sauna, it would just make the humidity more oppressive. I wrote long letters home. From my dorm room, I could watch the Fulani tribesmen herding their scrawny cattle through the fields beside the hospital where I cared for dying babies.

In the afternoons, I analyzed the level of alpha-1-antitrypsin in the breast milk of healthy Nigerian mothers. This was, after all, a research program. When I went back to Pitt, I wanted to have something to show for it. We published our results in the *East African Medical Journal*,[54] and I won an award from the Allegheny County Medical Society. For doing *research*.

Infant mortality was high. The causes were absurdly preventable. Measles, diarrhea, diphtheria. There was tension between the modern doctors in the hospitals, who wanted to set up immunization programs, and the traditional healers, who reportedly delivered babies at home, cut their umbilical cords with a rusty knife, and dressed the wounds with spider webs. The Nigerian doctors I worked with were from the villages, but they had been educated in Europe and the United States and had come back with the firm convictions of any religious convert.

My time in Nigeria shaped my career, but not in straightforward ways. I saw how pitifully easy it would be to save lives. I realized that, if my goal as a doctor was simply to save as many lives as I could, I should leave the United States and go almost anywhere else. There was no magic to it and not much skill. With a backpack full of tetanus toxoid or oral rehydration solution, I could trek through most countries in the world and save more lives in a week than I would save in Pittsburgh or Chicago in my entire lifetime. For the cost of one student's tuition for a year at an American medical school, I could probably save a thousand lives. Conversely, if I did not do that, if I stayed in the United States, then my goal must be something else. Was that what Ken had sent me there to learn?

Why did Ken refuse a liver transplant? Was that part of the lesson he was trying to teach? That saving lives is easy, but that living a life is much harder, and that medicine ought to be as much about the way we live our lives as it is about whether or not we can or should save lives?

I heard about Ken's death when I went to Pittsburgh to attend a big bioethics meeting. The meeting was unprecedented. Four national bioethics organizations had agreed to meet together, just once. Until that time, the four groups had guarded their identities and their separate national meetings as zealously as any warlord ever guarded a strategic hilltop hamlet. But that one year they met together to grapple with the major moral dilemmas of the day. I still wonder how they decided to divide the registration fees. Was there an ethics committee?

When I picked up my ID badge, I overheard a discussion among some registrants who had noticed that the badges for men had clips and the badges for women had pins. Why? Clearly, women's clothing is different, in significant ways, from men's, and the differences might justify this arcane form of gender discrimination. Men generally have a collar or a pocket; women generally have an uninterrupted expanse of cloth. That difference seems to favor giving the women pins and men clips, yet it seemed acceptable simply that the tags were different. It showed a laudatory attention to detail. Still, one registrant said that the policy decisions that were reached seemed a little inappropriate. Overhearing this conversation, I wondered what would happen when we got to the tougher moral issues.

A brief glance at the conference schedule showed that there would be plenty of tougher issues. There were workshops on euthanasia, sex selection, rationing, futility, health care reform, medical humanities, fiction, theater, movies. There were sessions addressing the special issues of Orthodox Jews, women, Norwegians, and "non-heart-beating cadavers." Now, one might think it unnecessary or redundant to specify that cadavers did not have beating hearts. Cadavers, after all, are dead, and thus we might expect that their hearts had stopped. However, in these troubled times, there are two definitions of death: the traditional, cardiorespiratory definition, which focuses on the irreversible cessation of heartbeat and breathing; and the neurologic definition ("brain death"), which focuses on the irreversible cessation of brain function. The hearts of brain-dead persons still beat; those of cardiologically dead persons do not.

The circumlocution of "non-heart-beating cadavers" is one of the many neologisms that have arisen as we try to come to grips with the implications of new ways of thinking about death. This particular semantic construction says much about the way bioethics has been changing the way we talk. The newly dead have taken on new significance as a result of the phenomenal success of organ transplantation. There are many more people waiting for organs than there are organs available. Transplant programs around the country are trying many different ways to increase the supply of organs without decreasing public support for transplantation. The concept of "brain death" was developed by medical experts in the late 1960s, in part to facilitate the retrieval of organs from people who didn't meet traditional criteria for death—that is, people whose hearts were still beating.

Brain death, defined as "the irreversible cessation of all brain function," has been widely accepted by most doctors, lawyers, and philosophers as being legally and morally equivalent to death. It has become something of a crusade among believers to ensure that society accepts the moral (and even biological) equivalence of "death" and "brain death." Dissenters who question this equivalence are thought of with the same disdain as people who question evolution and want to teach their children creationism.

As with any social movement, of course, there have been backlashes. Cultural consensus requires constant vigilance. New Jersey now allows a religious exemption to brain death for some Orthodox Jews who insist on a more traditional definition of death, which requires the cessation of breathing and heartbeat. This exemption leads to the interesting possibility that a last-minute conversion to Orthodox Judaism or a trip across the Delaware from Philadelphia to Camden could bring a dead man back to life. Wonder of wonder, miracle of miracles!

I was happy to get back to Pittsburgh. I had graduated from the University of Pittsburgh School of Medicine in 1981 and had been back only rarely since. The bioethics meeting was held shortly after two big USAir plane crashes. Many attendees agonized over which airline to fly to Pittsburgh. Analyses of the accidents showed no real patterns, no smoking gun. Statisticians from Harvard were quoted in *USA Today* as saying that you could get on a plane once a day for the next twenty-six thousand years before, statistically speaking, you'd be in a crash. Tell me about it. I chose to fly American.

The big event of the first day of the megameeting was a discussion of medical futility. Medical futility has been a prominent topic in bioethics and health policy, but of all the issues floating around the bioethics world, the debate about medical futility has been one of the most difficult to explain to the uninitiated. Unlike euthanasia or surrogate mothers or the use of growth hormone therapy to make short kids taller, all of which seem to be issues that ordinary citizens can grasp, the debate over medical futility seems to remain opaque or amorphous. It is hard for people to zero in on the fundamental values that are at stake. People talk past one another. This suggests to me that the really important issues in the futility debate are being cloaked, rather than illuminated, by the terms in which the debate has taken place.

The futility debate has been posed in one of two ways. One way is to ask whether doctors have a moral obligation to offer patients useless, or futile, treatments simply because the patients say they want such treatments. Stated this way, it seems to be a question of whether patients have an absolute entitlement to squander vast amounts of societal resources arbitrarily and to force physicians' complicity in an absurd enactment of their irrational whims. Any reasonable person would say they do not have such a right. In other words, framed in this way, the debate is over before it has begun.

Another formulation of the futility debate is to ask whether doctors may decide, using their own idiosyncratic personal values, whether the benefits of a particular treatment are so low (or the costs so high) that the treatment should not even be offered to a patient, or whether, by contrast, the patient's perceptions and values are necessarily a part of the decision-making process. Framed in this way, many reasonable people would argue that physicians do not have the right to impose their own or even perceived societal values on patients, and that if they are given this right, it will be the end of patient autonomy and informed consent—the beginning of a long slide down a slippery slope toward a type of physician paternalism that is no longer acceptable or desirable.

The debate has come to a head in a number of particular cases. One case involved a baby (dubbed "Baby L" by the courts) in Boston who had severe brain damage. She was blind, deaf, and quadriplegic.

Because she couldn't swallow, she had multiple episodes of aspiration pneumonia and had been in the intensive care unit on a ventilator many times. At one point her doctors decided that continued aggressive treatment was both futile and inhumane. They told her mother that they refused to put her back on a ventilator. Her mother insisted otherwise and took the case to court.[55]

The mother of Baby L had agreed to come to the bioethics meeting in Pittsburgh to present her side of the story, and the Kings Garden Conference Room of the Pittsburgh Hilton, where the futility session was being held, was packed. The session turned nasty. An ethicist who had written an article about Baby L in the *New England Journal of Medicine* got into a heated argument with Baby L's mother. She defended her decision to insist on continued treatment, saying that when the baby wasn't sick, she enjoyed life. The ethicist hoped to persuade her that it was morally unjustifiable to expend enormous amounts of societal resources to keep her chronically ill, multiply handicapped baby alive. She wouldn't agree. He pressed his point harder and harder, hoping to force her logically to acknowledge that her position was incompatible with justice in a system that had limited resources. She wanted him to see that justice doesn't apply to decisions a mother makes for her daughter.

Many of the people in the room had agreed, in private and in the abstract, that Baby L should not have been put on a ventilator. Yet many were troubled and embarrassed by the direct confrontation with Baby L's mother in a public forum. She was an impressive, tall, handsome, African American, and there weren't too many other African Americans at the megameeting. She was soft-spoken but quite firm, and it was clear from the start that her position was not going to be changed by the clever, casuistic arguments of an ethicist. She believed in what she was doing from the bottom of her soul.

Afterward, one woman who witnessed the argument told me, "I was very upset. She was brave to come here and shouldn't have been humiliated like that. I should have spoken up and defended her." The woman looked ashamed, although I couldn't tell whether it was for her own moral failing in not speaking up or a larger shame at the difference between her responses to an abstract moral argument about futility and her responses to a wrenching human confrontation about a mother and child.

Things always seem simpler, somehow, in the abstract. Yet, it seemed as if many people may have changed their minds about futility as a result of seeing the particular mother of a particular baby. They learned something different. The case was about justice and resource allocation, but it was also about courage and love.

One of the perennial problems with medical education is that there is too much to learn. Generations of reformers have criticized the fact that there is too much memorization. Ironically, one of the terms used to describe memorization is learning "by heart." In fact, memorization is precisely the opposite: it is learning by brain, not by heart.

David Kirp recently wrote a book called *Learning by Heart: AIDS and Schoolchildren in America's Communities.*[56] It tells the stories of different communities trying to understand and make decisions about the first children in their schools who had AIDS, whether to welcome them in the schools or to exclude them. The dilemmas occurred again and again across the country, in small towns like Kokomo, Indiana, and Swansea, Massachusetts, and in big cities like New York and Chicago. Each responded differently. Some were generous and compassionate; others paranoid and self-protective. But the interesting thing is that each community had to learn how to do things itself. Neither the rules of the Centers for Disease Control (CDC) and the state health department nor the stories of other communities that appeared in the press really prepared people. You couldn't memorize the response; you had to experience it. It wasn't something objective and external; it was something that people had to live. They had to learn by their own hearts. These two different types of "learning by heart" seem crucial to understanding the problems of medical education, where there is too much memorization and too little compassion, too much knowledge and not enough understanding. It is a simpler matter to mold minds and to test whether they have been molded than to learn by heart.

I took some time off during the bioethics megameeting to cruise the halls of my old medical school. It was the first time I'd been back since graduation. I was astounded. There were new buildings everywhere. New research labs, a new children's hospital, new parking lots, a new cafeteria, new bridges connecting buildings between new upper stories that didn't even exist when I was there. Academic medical centers are always complaining that times are tough, that the fiscal strings are tightening, that their future is in jeopardy, but somehow they keep adding buildings at a steady clip. Pittsburgh's building spree seemed unprecedented, even by the inflated standards of American academic medical centers. I asked where all the money and energy had come from for this building craze. I got two answers: Starzl and Detre.

Dr. Thomas Starzl arrived in Pittsburgh the year I left, and had turned Pittsburgh into the transplant capital of the world. Patients and doctors from every country on earth came to Pittsburgh to be a part of the newest, most exciting, sexiest enterprise that medicine had to offer in the 1980s. Livers, kidneys, hearts, heart-lungs, intestinal transplants, they did it all. The hospital was filled with patients awaiting transplants or recovering from postoperative complications. The subspecialists in Pittsburgh all became experts in the rare and exotic complications associated with transplants: the opportunistic infections, the toxicities of the immunosuppressants. It was a great place to study iatrogenic disease. And it was good for the bottom line. Patients paid for their transplants up front.

Dr. Tomas Detre is perhaps less well known. A psychiatrist, he built a research empire at the Western Psychiatric Institute and Clinic and then went on to become vice-chancellor of the university. Long before many other deans or chancellors caught on, he realized that an academic medical center had to be run like the business enterprise that it was. Faculty had to produce revenue, either by seeing patients or by getting grants. Academic medical centers couldn't compete with most community hospitals on the clinical side, so the measure of excellence became grants, especially federal grants, with their lucrative indirect-cost ratios. Faculty who got grants thrived. The Medical Center became a grant-supported research factory. This, of course, is no different from what would go on at most major academic medical centers. It was part of a larger market mentality that was sweeping the country, a mentality that saw the creation of markets as a moral imperative, and the discipline of market forces as a benevolent, uplifting thing. By this view, hospitals would be better, in every sense, if they were forced to compete with other hospitals in the health care delivery market, and academic research would be better if it was forced to compete with biotech firms in the research and development market. Graduate students began to send their theses to the patent office before they would publish them.

Working my way through the maze of new corridors and research labs, I finally found my way to some hallways that I recognized. The old lecture rooms where I had sat for endless hours of anatomy, histology, and physiology. The distinctive smell of the lecture halls brought back memories of Nicholas Cauna, our anatomy professor, drawing diagrams of the pelvis or the brachial plexus on the board with colored chalk. I remembered the cockiness with which we had sat in the back, reading the *New York Times* or just dozing off, knowing that the note service would bring us the outline of the lecture by the next day. The most surprising smell was the acrid whiff of formaldehyde from the anatomy lab next door. I remembered my cadaver—the bumbling dissection, that smell that I could never quite wash off my fingers—and I wondered why the cadaver ritual persists in an age of 3-D computer reconstructions of any internal organ. Perhaps there is still no substitute for the feeling of dissecting a cadaver, for seeing a dead body.

In spite of all the changes, the new buildings, the new research labs, the fact that the hospital was filled with patients getting treatments that nobody had heard of when I was there, and suffering from complications of those treatments that nobody had even imagined when I was there, the anatomy lab stayed the same, the educational process seemed rooted in a tradition as old as Koch and Virchow and Pasteur.

But no, people told me, things were changing. There was a new curriculum. After a five-year planning process, it was finally being implemented. Curricular reform had not been easy. There were tough negotiations, political factions had dug in on a number of issues. None had worked so doggedly or effectively to bring about reform as Ken Schuit, who unfortunately hadn't lived to see it implemented.

That was the first I'd heard about Ken's death. I was shocked. I asked how he had died. A sad story, they said. A hushed silence followed.

Averted eyes. I persisted. Liver failure, they said. Fulminant hepatitis. Well, maybe cirrhosis. It turned out that Ken drank a bit. Nobody wanted to talk about it.

Ken's background was in anatomy. He had started his career with cadavers. After getting a Ph.D. and teaching anatomy for a while, he went to medical school, and then on to a fellowship in pediatric infectious disease. He did some good lab work, early in his career, on chemotaxis and phagocytes, but his research efforts lagged. He seemed more motivated by a desire to treat the simple diseases that we know how to treat—diarrhea, pneumonia, meningitis, malaria—than by the desire to discover new knowledge. That simple value choice made him a pariah in the modern medical center. There was no money in diarrhea.

Ken hated what was going on in tertiary care and in medical education. He got angry at students who knew more about graft-versus-host disease than about meningitis, or who were better at inserting an umbilical artery catheter into a 600-gram preemie than they were at talking to parents about the problems their child was having at school. But he also knew that it was not the students' fault. He was much more angry at his colleagues. When he was on the Infectious Disease consult service, he refused to take medical students to see consultations about patients with liver transplants or bone-marrow transplants because he didn't think that that was the sort of knowledge that medical students needed. This approach baffled his collegues, for whom those were the most interesting cases, interesting and bizarre pathology that we created ourselves.

Eventually, his enmity toward transplants and all that they were doing to the academic medical center and to medical education turned into a more generalized concern about the dark side of medical progress. He abandoned his rat models of phagocyte function and helped set up the medical student exchange program with the University of Benin. He visited West Africa many times and did some clinical studies on Respiratory Syncitial Virus infections in Benin City. Mostly, though, he became more interested in teaching and less interested in writing.

There were no good models for teaching students something other than the latest facts, so he had to make it up as he went along. He taught in a different way. Instead of stressing facts, he stressed skills and simple virtues. He taught us to take careful histories. That required good listening. And he taught that by being a good listener himself. He stressed thorough physical examinations and careful documentation in chart notes. He read every note that every student wrote, and critiqued the notes. He wanted people to speak and write clearly. He went over case presentations on rounds.

He thought that a good doctor should be available when patients needed someone to talk to or had questions to ask. He didn't lecture about it. He modeled it. He was always available for students, and was willing to talk to them about whatever was on their minds, about their lives, about their patients, about their problems. He didn't tell us what it meant to be committed to a caring and helping profession; he showed us. Teaching became the model for doctoring.

He was not an easy teacher. He demanded a lot. He didn't play favorites. But he recognized that caring for others is the essence of teaching, and that it is a difficult thing to do. He worked long hours. He didn't have much to go home to. Since a divorce in the early eighties, he had lived alone. His children didn't visit often. He had few friends in the medical center. His private life was very private. He seemed tuned in to the suffering of others but was unable to tell anybody about his own. Perhaps he was trying to train the sort of doctors whom he could imagine might some day be able to take care of him, who would start their inquiries with a man's suffering rather than with his disease. But he didn't quite succeed. Maybe he just ran out of time. Nobody knew he had a drinking problem until he collapsed in the cafeteria one day. In the ER, they noticed that he was slightly jaundiced.

In *The Plague,* Camus describes a priest, Paneloux, who struggles to understand how we should respond to the suffering that seems inevitable and ubiquitous in the world God created. Should we merely accept the plague? Should we stuggle against it? How could we both affirm God's will and, at the same time, affirm our freedom?

> There was no question of not taking precautions to comply with the orders wisely promulgated for the public weal in the disorders of a pestilence. Nor should we listen to certain moralists who told us to

sink on our knees and give up the struggle. No, we should go forward, groping our way through the darkness, stumbling perhaps at
times, and try to do what good lay in our power. As for the rest, we
must hold fast, trusting in the divine goodness, even as to the deaths
of little children, and not seeking personal respite.[57]

When Paneloux became ill, he refused to call for the doctor, clinging
instead to his crucifix. Ken also refused to call the doctor, and died alone
in a hospital bed. It is unclear whether he had anything at all to which
he could cling. Although his father had been a missionary, Ken had long
ago lost his own faith in religion.

Medical education is a problematic endeavor. Master physicians have
always been showmen, and there is a long tradition by which teaching is
accomplished through demonstrating how little students know. The grisly traditional rituals of teaching rounds involve a process, known as
"pimping," by which senior attending physicians question the students
until an area of ignorance is uncovered.[58] The students can never know
enough because there is an infinite amount to know. These teaching rituals have a strong central element of institutionalized sadism. One
famous professor of medicine at Pittsburgh used to pride himself on
making the students feel so stupid that they would cry.

Teaching is also the last activity in the academic medical center that
has not been "costed out." Medical students pay tuition, but that tuition
disappears into a vast budgetary maw and nobody knows where exactly
it goes. Academic medical centers receive bonus payments from
Medicare, which are supposed to support the extra costs of teaching, but
those are similarly difficult to account for precisely. Interestingly, this is
not a world without accountants. Every aspirin tablet, every endoscopy,
and every moment of a physician's time with patients has a precise price.
But not teaching. It remains either sacred, or devalued, depending on
one's point of view. Steven Shea and his colleagues recently argued in
the *New England Journal of Medicine* that teaching is astonishingly
devalued in medical schools, and that this situation is likely to get
worse.[59] They estimated that the compensation for teaching at Columbia
University Medical Center was about sixteen dollars an hour. In an

accompanying editorial, Jerome Kassirer, the editor of the journal, admits that changes in the financing of academic medical centers threaten their educational mission, but says that teaching "has its own intrinsic reward."[60] So does doctoring, but it's nice to get paid as well.

The relationship between teacher and student is like the relationship between doctor and patient. The teacher cares for the student, and knows more. The student must trust the teacher and do what the teacher asks, even if it seems painful or arcane or meaningless. The student must believe that the course of treatment will lead to desired results. Educators often treat students with the same mixture of superiority and aloofness that doctors bring to encounters with patients. Medical students seldom experience illness and the patient role, and so the student role is as close as they may get to seeing how different doctors care for others. The general lesson seems to be that we care only in the most cerebral way. Facts, not emotions, are the ultimate reality. We don't learn anything by heart.

Ken's approach was different. Instead of trying to show how little we knew, he helped us get better at what we were doing. He didn't seem to glorify himself by belittling us but instead saw our achievements and accomplishments as his own. Teachers, like doctors, must dance with the paradox that the better they are at what they do, the more invisible they will become. Students of the best teachers feel that they learned everything by themselves or discovered it for the first time. Patients of the best doctors feel that they were not that sick to start with.

Or at least that's the way it used to be. But today's doctors like to take responsibility for healing. They like to see the patient as the passive material upon which the doctor works his or her art, the block of marble that is chiseled into sculpture. For this view, surgery is the model. The patient, etherized upon the table, is cured when the surgeon's knife opens the patient's body and removes the disease. As in the prime-time television medical dramas, the central character is the doctor, not the patient.

Walker Percy, a physician and novelist, writes about physicians who practice a different way. They are neither surgeons nor scientists, nor are they particularly virtuous. Instead, Percy heroes are often clownlike, in jail or in disgrace, and they are contrasted with the successful, high-powered subspecialists, surgeons, or National Institutes of Health researchers. The mainstream medical enterprise, in Percy's vision, has become morally neutral or even morally suspect, but the physician is still a compelling figure as one who can make moral struggles against mainstream medicine and the successful physicians of the time.

In this view, the morality of medicine has become something separate from the moral struggle of the physician, and yet the physician's power is still recognized as crucial for carrying on the struggle. This reflects what philosopher Jacob Needleman writes in *The Way of the Physician:* "All that the calling of the physician has represented throughout the centuries has vanished from view. It still exists, this calling, but it has retreated into the realm of the invisible, waiting for real men and women to allow its reappearance." As a result, "the doctor of today is either riddled with tension or stuffed with complacency. But above and beyond this, he is bored. He is nervous and bored or complacent and bored."[61] Bored with the mundane aspects of illness, disease, and treatment, and addicted to the adrenaline rush of innovation, of discovering even more new and dangerous approaches to therapeutics, and adhering to a weird, radical utilitarianism, by which money spent on medicine becomes a symbolic commitment to a warped humanism that justifies palaces built in honor of medical science in the burned-out killing fields of our inner cities. We can treat extreme prematurity but cannot prevent it, can save the gunshot-wound victim but cannot protect him, can ventilate and dialyze the octogenarian but cannot provide home health aides to bathe her. And we see these irrationalities as temporary by-products of a millenarian vision in which someday, soon, through gene therapy or advances in molecular biology, there will be no more premature babies, violence, or debilitated octogenarians. Or we see them as exemplary, as a new and better way of caring and of healing.

Part of the drive has been economic. From the perspective of hospital budgets, the best treatments have been those that require long and intense hospitalizations: heart surgery, transplantation, cancer chemotherapy, neonatal intensive care. In these cases, one needs lots of technology, lots of people, and lots of money, and it all goes toward intervention in a crisis for an identifiable patient. The sicker the patient, or the sicker we can make her or him, the more justifiable the expenditure. Subtle, preventive treatments don't capture our imaginations, don't commandeer the same resources, and those who provide such treatments are thus much more peripheral to this modern medical enterprise.

Ken was able to help others but was not able to ask for help himself. He lived alone. There were rumors about his private life. He drank. The more desperate he became, the better he became as a teacher. Had his work been recognized, things might have been different. He needed to get something back. Unfortunately, there is no place for such a teacher in today's medical center, just as there may be no place for the kind of doctors he was trying to teach in today's health care system. If he was depressed, it was more of a spiritual or philosophic depression than a psychiatric depression, like Paneloux in *The Plague* or Virginia Woolf when the war broke out. From a career perspective, teaching in today's academic medical center is a suicidal gesture. But it is also an affirmation that today's academic medical center may not be the best of all possible worlds, that something very crucial is missing at the center. This is not a matter of technique; it is a matter of courage. We don't need more information, we need more commitment.

The most troubling clinical situations are those in which a patient has a set of goals or values different from the doctor's. Sometimes, as in Ken's case, patients refuse treatments that seem to be clearly beneficial. At other times, they insist on treatments that are unlikely to be of benefit. The two situations share an underlying theme. In both, patients are asking doctors for something that the doctors think is not proper, something unacceptable or even immoral. The patient wants to write a different script, to imagine a different sort of doctor, to reverse the power roles and force the doctor into silent complicity. Some such patient requests may be immoral, but to make such judgments seems to require a more robust view of the intrinsic morality of medicine than we now share.

At the University of Chicago, we sometimes ask our first-year medical students to write an oath, a set of vows to which they might bind themselves by a promise. They study other oaths and the commentaries upon them, they pick and choose among the deities to whom they might offer their promise, they argue about whether to accept or reject certain obligations. The exercise of trying to find a common morality is interesting. Perhaps the most interesting part is that they can never agree on much. No two students are willing to be bound by precisely the same principles. The center has long since ceased to hold.

I'm not sure I could write an oath that would embody the morality of the medical profession, any more than I could write one that would embody the morality of teaching. It may be that an oath is the wrong format for such describing morality. A eulogy might be better. Vague promises are easy, but life may demand things of us for which we never prepared. Our lives themselves, more than the words, become an embodiment of the promises we make, and we don't know whether we've kept them until life is over.

Pornography has been famously characterized as something that we can't define but we know it when we see it. Morality may be something that we can't define but we know it when it's gone, when somebody who has it dies and we suddenly realize how how much poorer and emptier the world can seem in ways that we didn't appreciate when the somebody was there and filled our world with a sort of energy, with a sort of resistance, with a sort of strength.

6

Truths, Stories, Fictions, and Lies

Truth telling, in medicine, is a peculiar cultural practice. In the United States, doctors seem to endorse it more than doctors in most other places, and we endorse it more strongly today than ever before. It seems to play a central role in our conception of the proper relationship between patients and doctors. Any deviation from a standard of total honesty is seen as a doctor's way of preserving paternalistic power over patients. Truth telling is thus seen as necessary for patient empowerment, and patient empowerment is seen as an essentially good thing. We strive to demystify illness and imagine that truth is the first step toward clarity without supernaturalism.

Truly, we are a truth-crazed society. We strongly believe that there are truths out there in the world waiting to be discovered and that when we discover them, the knowledge will empower us and set us free. This way of approaching the issue of truth telling is as American as apple pie. It imagines a fundamentally exploitative relationship between the empowered and the disempowered and an overarching set of rational rules that we hope will level the playing field and help the disempowered avoid abuse. We are so used to this way of thinking about things that it is hard to see it as parochial, culture-bound, or idiosyncratic.

Carl Elliot is a bioethicist from South Carolina, now living in Montreal, who has spent a lot of time in other countries: Germany, Scotland, New

Zealand, South Africa. He has written about how hard it is to explain to foreigners the peculiar twists and turns of American bioethics, the focus on individualism, autonomy, privacy, the suspicion of authority. He writes:

> I have found that non-Americans occasionally find it difficult to understand all the fuss over the "right to die" debate in America, and the vehemence with which it is sometimes argued. Why would anyone want to continue treating a patient in a persistent vegetative state with virtually no chance of recovery? Ah, well, I usually explain, you must also understand how the right to die is related to the right to life, and to the debate over abortion, and to American churches, and to the role of the church in small-town life; you must also understand something about American hospitals, and feminism and libertarianism and fundamentalism and natural rights and John Locke and Thomas Jefferson and so on and so on ad infinitum.[62]

Following Jacques Barzun, he concludes that ethics is so embedded in culture that to understand American bioethics, you have to understand baseball.

A recent case on the Medical College of Wisconsin Bioethics Discussion Forum on the Internet raised a conflict about truth telling and about the peculiarities of our modern American approach to such dilemmas. Here was the case:

> A 9-year old girl with AIDS has developed chronic lung disease and AIDS nephropathy. Her lung disease is progressive but she does not yet require supplemental oxygen. Her kidney function is less than 20% of normal and continuing to decline. It is likely that she will require dialysis within the next year if she does not die from other complications of AIDS sooner. She is receiving total parenteral nutrition through a central intravenous line.
>
> The patient is aware that she has a chronic illness but not that she has AIDS. But she wonders about it. When she asked her mother whether she had AIDS, her mother responded "No."
>
> The mother also has AIDS (the patient's AIDS was perinatally transmitted). She (the mother) is quite ill and likely to die before the patient. In a recent discussion, she told the doctors that she would

like to tell her daughter that she (the daughter) has AIDS. However, the patient's grandmother is adamant that the 9-year-old not be told. So far this request is being respected by both her mother and the professionals.

The attending physician strongly believes that the patient should be told of her diagnosis. As stated above, the patient is already suspicious. The attending feels that continued concealment of information will be particularly harmful if/when the patient eventually finds out her diagnosis. The setting is a teaching hospital, with many consultants, students, residents, and support services involved. Someone will likely reveal the information to the patient, if only inadvertently, if she is an inpatient for a long enough time.[63]

The question put to an international cyberethics community was whether the doctors should continue to honor the grandmother's wishes that the nine-year-old not be told that she has AIDS.

Well, what is this case about? On one level, it is a simple question about truth telling. Most people believe that it is a good thing to tell the truth. We learned that one in kindergarten. Honesty is the best policy and so on. And yet, in both real life and in medical ethics, the distinction between truth telling and lying seems a little too stark and dichotomous. After all, we also teach our kindergartners to say they're sorry even if they're not really sorry, to tell grandma they loved her present even if they didn't, to be nice to kids in their class even if they don't like them. We want them to tell the truth but to judge how much of the truth, and to whom, and for what purpose. We want honesty but also sensitivity, kindness, etiquette.

As doctors, we usually inform patients of some but not all of the risks of an antibiotic before we prescribe it, or some but not all of the things that a blood test might reveal before we order it. We may exaggerate the expected benefits of treatment if we want people to consent to it or exaggerate the harms if we do not. A certain amount of lying, or at least of hypocrisy, seems to be part of every child's moral education, a part of what it means to be a civilized human being, and certainly a part of what it means to be a doctor.

I recently testified in a child abuse case, where I swore to tell the truth, the whole truth, and nothing but the truth. I was then asked a series of deceitfully misleading questions by lawyers on both sides. In some cases, it was impossible to answer the question without conveying views that I thought mangled the truth. Nobody asked me questions that got at what I thought was the whole truth. It was like being asked, "Have you stopped beating your wife?" and told to give only a yes or no answer. Either answer will be false. Silence might be best.

Silence, that is, a lie of omission, is generally easier to justify than uttering outright falsehoods. Here, also, conventional wisdom helps us out. "If you don't have anything nice to say," our kindergarten teachers admonished us, "then don't say anything at all." This aphorism embodies serious moral contradictions that are seldom acknowledged. A rigorous moral standard of honesty seems to demand that we say what is true whether it is nice or not. The admirable sentiment that kindness ought to preempt honesty is, on one level, an exhortation to dissemble.

In medicine, of course, there is a long and distinguished tradition of lying. In his book *The Silent World of Doctor and Patient,* J. Katz shows that from the time of Hippocrates until the late twentieth century, doctors not only routinely withheld the truth from patients but also vigorously defended the morality of their decisions to do so.[64] The arguments for withholding the truth varied. Some were patient-centered, claiming that the truth might be too difficult to bear. "Reassure the patient and declare his safety, even though you may not be certain of it," wrote Isaac Israeli, a ninth-century physician, "for by this you will strengthen his Nature." Other arguments focused on the physician and his moral obligation to foster hope. Thomas Percival, writing in the late eighteenth century, counseled doctors, "The physician should be the minister of hope and comfort to the sick." Some of the arguments were economic, that doctors who admitted uncertainty would frighten and discourage patients, and would soon go out of business. But none of the arguments were apologetic. Following this ancient moral tradition, doctors learned to withhold potentially stressful information, to conceal bleak diagnoses, and not to discuss the risks of treatments or procedures. In doing so, they were following the moral maxim of either saying nice things or saying nothing at all.

In light of this history, recent moral sentiment that patients ought to be told the whole truth, no matter how horrible it might be or how ill-prepared they might be to hear it, represents one of those mysterious sea changes in morality that occur from time to time whereby something that was once thought intolerable rather suddenly comes to be thought of as obligatory. When we note such a moral shift, it is important to ask why it occurred. Generally, it will not be that morality itself has changed, so that what was wrong then is right now. Instead, circumstances change and people confront new situations for which the conventional moral wisdom may not be entirely applicable.

Truth Telling in Historical Context

I believe that four major changes in the way we practice medicine led to a reevaluation of the presumption that patients should be kept in the dark. First, doctors have a different sort of knowledge about their patients than doctors did in the past. In particular, doctors today may know that patients are sick before the patients know that they are sick. Patients who are diagnosed before they are sick are not really patients. They have not felt the physical symptoms that lead to the metaphysical dread and fear. People who are ill and suffering, who know pain and perceive their own mortality, are in a different psychological and metaphysical state than healthy people. Literature by patients or about sickness suggests that they exaggerate fears, crave reassurance, eschew rationality, and deify their doctors.[65] Denial, magical thinking, and a focus on the present rather than the future are all expected, and perhaps desirable, responses to news of serious illness.[66] Traditional medical ethics, which encouraged hopeful evasion of difficult truths, acknowledged the special psychological realities of the sick patient in a way that modern bioethics does not.

The healthy patient with an abnormal screening test is in a completely different position from the acutely ill patient. He or she comes to the doctor not as a patient in pain and fear, looking for reassurance and hope, but as a healthy person seeking the statistically likely reassurance of continued health. Medicine becomes less of a response to crisis and more of a consumer good that may affect the person's health, like smoke detectors or dual air bags. There is no question of denial or reassurance. Instead, the well person who must make a treatment decision for himself or herself may be able to effectuate that state of alienation that we call rationality and carefully evaluate the risks and benefits of different treatment options as items on a store shelf or cars in a showroom might be evaluated.

The second important change in medical practice that led to the need for informed consent was a change in the toxicity of our treatments. Many surgical and medical therapies initially make patients worse than the diseases they treat. Our interventions take patients who feel quite healthy and make them feel very sick in order to make them well again. The age-old medical adage to do no harm has become essentially obsolete in modern medicine. We do harm all the time, generally in hope of achieving a greater good.

Two of the earliest informed-consent malpractice cases involved such cases and led judges to conclude that doctors could no longer hide the facts from patients. In one, the physicians caring for Martin Salgo, a fifty-five-year-old man with cramping leg pains, recommended an aortogram. When Mr. Salgo awoke after the procedure, he could not move his legs, and he sued the doctors for negligently failing to warn him of the risks of paralysis inherent in the procedure. Mr. Salgo's claim was poignant because the doctors, although apparently not negligent in performing the procedure, made the patient worse than he was before he sought their help. In such situations, the judges thought, it was not justifiable to withhold information about toxicity.[67]

Similarly, in *Natanson v. Kline,* a patient suffered damage from radiation therapy given her after a mastectomy in order to prevent recurrence of her breast cancer.[68] She later sued her doctor for not warning her about the effects that radiation therapy would have on her. Again, this was a situation in which a patient suffered a foreseeable side effect of a therapy that had not been negligently delivered.

These situations are not unique to modern medicine. One could argue that they existed in the days of blood letting, amputation for gangrene, or the use of foxglove for dropsy. But they are both more common and more predictable today. Thus, they create an obligation for truth telling that may not have existed before.

A third, related change has to do with the sophistication of our clinical epidemiological data that creates choices among different therapies with quantifiable outcomes for each. The pressures ensuing from the development of clinical epidemiology drive us toward shared decision making. To the extent that we study and compare the effectiveness and the side effects of treatments, we know with some precision how well they might work and what the risks of each might be.

Once we have quantified both the benefits and the side effects of treatments, it becomes clear that in many cases there is no longer one therapy that is clearly the "best" treatment. We see this in all areas of medicine. Decisions among different treatments for the same disease often incorporate nonclinical values. For example, different treatments for laryngeal cancer may offer different outcomes in terms of five-year survival, ability to speak, and ability to swallow. Different treatments for prostatic hypertrophy might offer different outcomes in terms of incontinence, urinary retention, impotence, or likelihood of developing cancer. The existence of well-defined choices creates challenges for doctors and patients, both of whom want to know what is "best." In such situations, the term *best* is necessarily value-laden. There is often no "best" treatment unless *best* is further defined. We must ask, "Best in terms of what?" Because any determination of what is best must include both clinical data and the patient's values, the patient must be informed of the options and participate in decision making.

The final change is the incorporation of a progressive mentality into medicine. Both doctors and patients today think of medicine as an enterprise in which progress will be continuous and inexorable. We expect treatment to get better, life expectancy to increase, infant mortality to fall. To further that progress, we understand that new therapies will be continuously introduced and evaluated.

The existence of a research agenda creates moral problems for clinical investigators and their patients. Patients want the latest treatments but don't want to be experimented upon. Investigators need to determine what is safe and effective, but don't want to compromise their loyalty to patients. One solution to this problem has been to develop ethical guidelines for research. The central ethical principle is that patients must be

informed when they are participating in research, must be told the risks
and benefits of the research project to them, and must be free to with-
draw at any time. These guidelines for clinical research have helped
create a climate in which information is more readily shared among doctors and patients.

It must be acknowledged that in general the movement toward truth
telling in medicine has come about mostly because of pressure from
lawyers and judges, that is, the standard was imposed on medicine from
the outside through a series of malpractice cases. These cases were but-
tressed by moral arguments that asserted that patients, like all citizens,
had a right to make autonomous decisions and that they needed information that only doctors could provide in order to make those decisions.
Doctors initially howled in protest at the new, legally imposed standard
for communication and truth telling. Even doctors engaged in clinical
research felt that discussing procedures in detail with patients was inappropriate. As recently as 1965, Donald Fredrickson, director of the
National Heart Institute, could oppose disclosure because it might
"unduly alarm the patient and hinder his reasonable evaluation of procedures important to his welfare."[69]

More recently, doctors have embraced the concept of informed consent. Unfortunately, this has not always been for reasons initially
imagined by judges and philosophers. The requirement that patients
give informed consent was initially thought to be a fundamental change
in the moral basis of the doctor-patient relationship. In particular, it was
seen as a way of allowing patients and doctors to share responsibility for
decision making, of reducing the silence that Katz abhorred, and of
equalizing the power balance between doctors and patients. In reality
today, it more often disempowers patients. In his recent novel *Operation
Wandering Soul*, Richard Powers describes a girl from Laos trying to
explain an informed consent form to her father, who speaks no English:
"If you want them to treat me, you must agree not to ask for lots of money
if they make a mistake and something bad happens."[70] Informed consent
is like the disclaimer on the back of a ski-lift ticket: "Surgery is a dangerous sport." If we tell patients about bad outcomes and they consent,
then they are responsible, not us. Rather than a way of sharing power,

truth telling and the process of seeking consent has become a way of evading accountability.

The goals of law and the goals of ethics are not the same. The law is better at defining minimally acceptable behavior and leads to the development of standards that represent the lowest common denominator of social acceptability. Fine distinctions are drawn between what is minimally acceptable and what is impermissible, rather than between what is good and what is excellent. This self-protective legal approach, rather than the more idealistic ethical approach, has shaped truth telling and informed consent in American medicine. This is not to blame the lawyers. Instead, responsibility lies with the doctors who do need heed moral critiques but will change their behavior in a minute in response to punishments meted out to their colleagues by judges or juries, and even then tend to do what they must rather than what they ought.

Informed Consent, Empowerment, and Pediatrics

As with most modern bioethical paradigms, all bets are off when it comes to pediatrics. Pediatrics highlights the differences between legal and moral obligations because, in general, our legal obligations are to the patient's legal guardian, but our moral obligations are to the patient (and perhaps to the guardian as well). Given this split, many of the rationales that I have outlined for the recent changes in moral views of truth telling in medicine do not readily apply to children. They are not empowered to make decisions or evaluate treatment options and so may not derive the practical benefits from information that adults derive. One response to this is the movement to empower children. For example, the American Academy of Pediatrics recently endorsed the concept that we must seek the child's "assent" to treatment and to participation in research.[71] This somewhat ambiguous concept is an important step toward acknowledging the ability of children to understand and to make decisions. Even those who most enthusiastically seek to empower children acknowledge, however, the limitation for the very young or very sick child, situations where we will continue to turn to the parents.

Nobody has dealt with the really hard case of what to do when a young child does not assent to a treatment that both doctors and parents feel is clearly in his or her best interest. If it is a good thing to tell children the truth in such cases, it is not for the same practical or operational reasons that we tell adults. Instead, arguments for truth telling must draw on a more pure moral ideal. We tell the truth to children, it seems, not to empower them, or to gain their cooperation and achieve good outcomes, or to make them aware of our conflicts of interest, but simply because the truth is good.

Interestingly, among all the responses to the case of the nine-year-old girl with HIV on the Internet, everybody seemed to take it for granted that she *ought* to be told the truth, and that her mother and grandmother were wrong not to tell her. Debate was less about that issue than it was about the role of the physician. Throughout the discussion that stretched out for weeks of learned arguments and counterarguments that were sometimes subtle, sometimes sublime, sometimes nuanced, and sometimes just stupid, there never seemed to be any doubt but that the truth was good and that ethicists and doctors both supported it. It was seen as unfortunate that we were limited in our ability to do good by a respect for family privacy and for the rights of parents to do things that are bad for their children as long as they are not too bad. The problem was thus conceptualized as one of deciding how to act when the world is less noble then we are.

None of the discussion focused on the particular issues associated with AIDS. There was the sense that the nature of that particular diagnosis should not be morally relevant, that the issue of truth telling was non-context-dependent. We should apply the same rules to disclosure of a diagnosis of HIV that we would apply to telling a nine-year-old that she has chicken pox or pneumonia or cancer. Yet, AIDS is different. Children get it from their parents. It is a stigmatizing illness. It is associated with homosexuality, intravenous drug use, and prostitution. These facts about AIDS, it seemed to me, were not morally neutral or irrelevant.

I found myself wondering whether our way of dichotomizing the choices was sufficient. In other words, do the two choices—to override the mother and grandmother and tell the girl the truth, or to respect family privacy grudgingly, even though we believe in our hearts that a disservice is being done to our patient—exhaust our moral imagination as we think about this case? Somehow, neither choice seemed satisfying. I didn't want to do either. It seemed that these views of both morality and truth telling were too thin, and that both were demeaning to the richer story that was playing itself out before us. We seemed to be focusing on the tiniest moral issues with a reductionism learned from the scientists, whose truths accrete bit by bit, in a way that ethical truths do not. It may be that this way of thinking is the only way to gain a voice in the world of the scientists. But the price for gaining such a voice may be too high.

Bioethics among the Scientists

I found myself worrying about "voice" when I was invited to address the bioethics session of the combined meetings of the Society for Pediatric Research, the American Pediatric Society, and the Ambulatory Pediatrics Association in Seattle a few years ago. At the meeting, thousands of pediatricians and scientists from around the world gathered to hear the latest news from research laborotories. There were papers on gene therapy, liquid ventilation, urban violence, and bed wetting. Some of the sessions seemed to be in a new language of abbreviations and acronyms. Papers were presented with titles like "Interferon alpha (IFNa) treatment of fulminant EBV-associated B-cell lymphoproliferative disease (BLPD) following T-cell depleted (T-D) haploidentical bone marrow transplantation (BMT)."

Although the meetings were primarily concerned with basic science, there was also a bioethics session. It focused mainly on issues of death and dying, and was attended by people who seemed to be wondering what we ought to do when all the interferon alpha (IFNa) in the world just won't help any more.

I was thrilled to be invited because, in addition to the honor, I got seventeen hundred frequent flier miles each way. Although the talk wasn't until Monday, I flew out on Saturday night to get the supersaver fare. For a thousand bucks, I'll spend another night away from my wife and kids.

To tell the truth, it wasn't just the money. My kids always ask me why I travel and I say that I hate it, it's part of my job, that I'd much rather be with them. Of course, I'm not being entirely honest. If I were, I might say that it's actually great to get away, to have a little time to myself with no schlepping to soccer practice, flute lessons, or Hebrew school. No stupid sibling rivalries to put up with. No dishes to do. And all on an expense account, albeit a frugal one. In Seattle, I had all day Sunday on my own, which was a good thing because I hadn't yet written my talk. Months before, when I was asked to speak, I had whimsically chosen the title "Does Bioethics Matter?" Now, I had to take a position.

I sat under a tree in Elliot Bay Park, watching the ferries periodically head out to the islands. The sun was out! I could see the mountains in the distance. I wrote, I read novels, I sipped cappuchino, which seemed worth it at the time but came back to haunt me that night. Even without coffee, I can't sleep well on the road. With coffee, forget it. After midnight, the hotel clocks slow down. When the air conditioner starts, I wake up. I hear the toilet flush in the room next door. The pillows aren't quite right.

I lay awake, going over my just-written talk in my head, reworking the conclusion, wondering whether people would laugh at my jokes and, if they did, whether they'd think I was just a clown. Old friends, colleagues, and teachers would all be there. Why, I wondered, did I pick such an amorphous topic at a meeting devoted to reductionist objectivism? I must have a will to fail. My heart started to race a little. Was this from too much coffee? Pretalk anxiety? Or a rare cardiac arrhythmia? Is this how it will end for me, a sudden cardiac arrest, alone in a nonsmoking room? How can it be? I don't deserve to die so young. I exercise, I eat a lot of fish. The fish! Maybe it's the sushi doing me in. Everything out there, especially the things that are good for you, are also dangerous. If I did die here, on the thirty-second floor of the Seattle Sheraton, I wondered who would find me, seventeen hundred frequent flier miles from those I love?

My wife doesn't like to travel and has a hard time when I do. She likes her house, her garden, her own bed. Its hard to explain the attraction of travel, the schmoozing, the excitement, the fertile interplay of ideas. But I find it good to get away. I had lunch with a woman I went out with during medical school. She talked about how tough it is do be a mom and start a career, about the special burdens career women still have. I empathized. We agreed that it was great to get away alone once in a while, to have time for leisurely lunches where nobody pages you and somebody else has to pick up the kids. She was at the meeting without her husband. I was there alone, too. We looked at the schedule of presentations for the afternoon, wondering together whether there was really anything worth hearing. Fertile interplay of ideas, indeed.

So there I lay, a professional moralist, sleepless in Seattle, the night before a major speech on the importance of ethics, thinking about adultery. I thought of changing the title of my talk to "Does Sin Matter?"

Well, once I started thinking of both death and sex, there was no use trying to get back to sleep. I turned on the light and started reading. In the airport on the way out, I had bought Peter Kramer's *Listening to Prozac*, which seemed like a good read for an insomniac having anxiety attacks. Kramer discusses how new psychoactive drugs not only alleviate the symptoms of anxiety disorders and obsessive-compulsive disorders but also seem to make people genuinely happy and more satisfied with their lives in a way that they never were before. Kramer's patients extricate themselves from abusive relationships, get along better with their children, work more productively, date nicer men, sleep better, lose weight. He wonders whether such outcomes are proper goals for medicine, whether they are the sorts of things doctors should be facilitating with drug treatment.[72]

We face similar dilemmas with drugs such as a growth hormone that makes short kids taller, drugs such as Ritalin that help kids who have trouble paying attention, drugs such as estrogen that treat and reverse the natural effects of aging. These problems are not diseases, although they may cause suffering. Is the goal of medicine to allow everybody to live happily, date nice men, play golf until we're a hundred, and then die quickly and peacefully? If so, shouldn't we be willing to finish people off at the end with a quick and painless injection?

They won't convict Dr. Kevorkian in Michigan. A number of federal courts have approved physician-assisted suicide. According to an Oregon law, "An adult who is capable, is a resident of Oregon, and has been determined by the attending physician and consulting physician to be suffering from a terminal disease, and who has voluntarily expressed his or her wish to die, may make a written request for medication for the purpose of ending his or her life in a humane and dignified manner in accordance with this Act."[73]

Euthanasia has been widely practiced in the Netherlands for a decade. I recently heard a neonatologist from Amsterdam talking about their approach to death and dying. He presented two cases. One involved a premature baby born after just six-and-a-half months of gestation. Like many premature babies, she suffered a massive brain hemorrhage leading to irreversible brain damage. Her parents and doctors agreed that her quality of life would be unacceptable and decided to stop the ventilator. She died quickly in her mother's arms. The second case involved a baby born after seven and a half months of gestation who also had a massive brain hemorrhage. It was clear that he would also have irreversible brain damage. They stopped his ventilator too, but he didn't die. Would it be acceptable, the Dutch doctor asked, not to put him back on the ventilator? To withhold antibiotics if he developed pneumonia? To withhold fluid or nutrition? To give morphine if he seemed to be in pain? To give a lethal injection? The doctor argued that a lethal injection would be the most humane way of achieving the goal that everyone sought, which was to allow the baby to die peacefully.

In this country, we would allow the ventilator to be stopped, and would allow medical treatment to be withheld. We can't decide whether fluid and nutrition should be considered a medical treatment in such a case. We might even allow morphine to be administered. But we would consider a lethal injection to be dangerously unethical and illegal. Even proponents of legalized euthanasia would limit it to competent adults. Are the Dutch doctors more humane than we are, or less? Are they going down the road that leads to eugenics and Nazi atrocities? They struggled against the Nazis, hid Anne Frank, and have a system of universal health coverage. Whatever slope they are going down, it seems a bit different from the one taken by the Nazis.

Well, I didn't get very far with *Listening to Prozac,* and I didn't get much sleep that night. I was still awake as the sun rose, so I headed out for a jog by the waterfront. At that hour, the mountains on the Seattle horizon seemed to float above the clouds. It was mystical, otherworldly. I inhaled the salty-fish smell from the bay and felt great. Who needs sleep, anyway? I love this life in the academic jet set.

A lot of other pediatricians were already out jogging. Most didn't look really happy. Just part of the job, some sort of medico-spiritual exercise. Keeping their risk factors down. The day before, I had seen a few pediatricians smoking in the alley outside the convention center. I certainly hope they're not in my insurance risk pool.

People argue about whether morality changes over time, whether the goal of ethical analysis should be to develop timeless moral principles. It seems to me that it does change. The evidence is all around us. It used to be that one could smoke cigarettes in hotel rooms but had to go out into a dark alley to buy pornography. Now, we can lie in bed and choose among four dirty movies on Spectravision but have to sneak out into the alley for a smoke.

I sidestepped a homeless man sleeping in a doorway, noticed a couple of hippies watching me disdainfully from a park bench. My Nikes pounded the pavement. Down by the waterfront, the rays of the morning sun lighted up a large sculpture: three smooth marble pedestals and three big blocks of granite. One block was on a pedestal, one was leaning against a pedestal, and one was on the ground beside a pedestal. It was called "Upon, Against, Adjacent."

Last year, my wife, a pediatrician, took time off from her job in an inner-city community health center to go to art school. She would paint all day and take espresso breaks with purple-haired, leather-clad, spike-necklaced art students who have lots of their body parts pierced. And she would come home in a state of spiritual turmoil. She loved to paint, but compared to the immediacy of teen pregnancy, child abuse, and counseling suicidal teenagers, painting seemed frivolous. She would ask, "Does art matter?" I was preparing for my trip to Seattle, and would respond, "Does bioethics matter?" Dinner table conversation often ground to a halt.

I looked at the sculpture again. Underneath the "adjacent" rock there was a homeless man sleeping. This art seemed to have found a purpose.

Bioethics never kept anybody out of the rain. So what, I wondered, were we doing at this research meeting, among the thousands of scientists who were working to cure genetic disease, to develop new drugs for the relief of human suffering, to save the lives of children? Were we really part of the team? Does what we do matter?

Doing the Right Thing

Increasingly, people are questioning the values and the presumptions of medicine, asking whether our way of caring for people is the best way. The administrative structure of medicine is being overhauled from top to bottom by governments, by market managers, by physician executives and health management consultants. At the same time, new advances in medical science promise a new era of biologic innovation, with everything from fetal surgery to gene therapy to treatments to prevent aging. Each innovation comes with a promise and a price, and the more we innovate, the more we are forced to question and compare and prioritize among interventions, populations, problems, and allocation schemes. The individualistic morality that sees virtue in the unencumbered and unswervingly loyal commitment of each doctor to each single patient seems to be crumbling under the assault. Medical societies agonize over the compromises that doctors are being forced to make. Journals are filled with soul-searching articles bemoaning the changes and looking for villains. We blame the corrupt government or the greedy managed care administrators or the heartless market.

Should doctors fight the trend to rethink the way we allocate health care resources, or should they welcome it as inevitable and potentially beneficial? Most doctors want to be moral, to do the right thing They think long and hard about the particular issues, such as in vitro fertilization, growth hormone for short kids, futile care for the demented elderly, euthanasia, genetic screening, health reform, and justice. Such thinking has created an international interest in bioethics, a movement with meetings in Milan, San Francisco, Paris, Amsterdam, and Buenos Aires. There are now at least six journals devoted to bioethics; there are home pages on the World Wide Web; there is even some government support for research in ethics.

In spite of the flurry of activity, it's hard to tell whether we're keeping up, whether we're getting more moral or even keeping our heads above water. There seems to be a creeping hollowness at the center of the hubbub. The more we see ethicists on the talk shows, ethicists in the *New York Times* and *Wall Street Journal,* ethicists in the courtroom, or ethicists making rounds in the intensive care unit, the more, it seems, we might properly ask what they're actually doing. What do the philosophers know that should allow them to make pronouncements about what is ethical?

Even among philosophers themselves, there is some skepticism about the usefulness of bioethics. Stephen Toulmin argues that medicine "saved the life of ethics" by bringing it back to a reality that in the mid-twentieth century, it had tried too hard to ignore.[74] "The central concerns of philosophers had become so abstract and general that they had, in effect, lost all touch with the concrete and particular issues that arise in actual practice, whether in medicine or elsewhere," he writes. "Once this demand for intelligent discussion of the ethical problems of medical practice and research obliged them to pay fresh attention to applied ethics, however, philosophers found their subject 'coming alive again' under their hands" (p. 749). Leon Kass argues that bioethicists focus too much on analysis of rare and exotic problems, and too little on the everyday action.[75] What has the bioethics movement done, he asks, to produce more virtuous physicians? George Annas argues that ethics has largely ignored the public policy aspect of medical resource allocation and so was unprepared to participate in the discussions of health reform.[76] All of these critics ask, in different ways, whether the bioethics movement has specific goals and whether they have been reached. In other words, how should we judge the goals, methods, aspirations, success, failure, or relevance of the entire enterprise?

In my talk for the researchers, I decided to focus on a recent book, *Raising Lazarus,* by Robert Pensack and Dwight Williams, a harrowing account of Pensack's life in medicine.[77] Pensack is a practicing psychiatrist in Colorado who was born with hypertrophic cardiomyopathy

(HCM), an autosomal dominant genetic condition that causes progressive heart failure. His mother died of it. He and his brother both have it. He tells of his memories of his mother's death, about how he and his brother were originally diagnosed, about how he almost died of the disease a number of times. His story is the weird modern tragedy of living with and coming to terms with one's genetic destiny, of being a loser in the genetic lottery, and of participating in the modern heroic epic of medical science's fight against genetic fate.

Pensack writes as both a patient and a doctor. He grew up at just the time when medical discoveries about his disease began to allow the possibility of treatment. Clinical trials of interventions for HCM were just starting at the National Institutes of Health when he was in medical school, and at the same time that his disease was relentlessly progressing. He is at the center in a maddeningly multifaceted way: studying about his disease, participating in the latest research studies, and literally trying to save himself.

He movingly presents the patient's perspective on innovative therapy, the uncertainties and the dashed hopes, the frustratingly impersonal doctors and the mistakes they make. He has vivid memories of the feeling as his heart starts to race in his chest and he falls to the floor in ventricular tachycardia. He gives an eerie account of an out-of-body experience at his own cardiac arrest, of his sense of hovering over the code team and watching his own electrocardiogram tape scroll out of the machine.

> At first there is terror, twirling colors, overwhelming claustrophobia, but I sense myself moving beyond that, beyond what I recognize as the phenomenal world into a peaceful country of shadows, an incomprehensible realm of sublime calm. The body—my body—floats, and as it does so I experience the ability to observe myself, the doctors and nurses in the laboratory where the electrocardiogram ushers out a ribbon of white paper with a steady black line on it. (pp. 120–21)

Pensack also has a doctor's perspective and tells how it feels to be both patient and doctor at the same time. Some of the experiences are macabre. While he is having a heart catheterization, he can feel the catheter and realizes that it is turning the wrong way inside his body. He tells the cardiologists but they ignore him, with the usual physician disdain for information from patients, until he screams that they should look at their screens and see where the catheter tip is. Sure enough, it is where he says it is, and they sheepishly pull it back.

His heart disease progresses to the point where his only hope is a transplant. He goes on the national waiting list and enters another lottery. This time, he's waiting along with hundreds of others for a young and healthy person with just the right blood type to die a violent death. Each day, he gets a little sicker. He carries a new kind of beeper, this one tuned to the transplant center. It goes off only when a heart becomes available. One time he is called, but it is a false alarm. The donor heart is no good. The waiting begins again, the beeper frighteningly silent.

In the end, Pensack gets a heart transplant. Postoperatively, he has numerous physical and mental complications, including a severe psychosis in which he imagines that his doctors are all CIA agents and that he is a Viet Cong spy they are trying to kill. There is a frightening lesson for us all in Pensack's detailed recounting of each episode, each complication, from the point of view of an observer who knows better than most patients can ever know what is being done to him and why. In spite of all that he knows, he is relentlessly dehumanized and literally driven crazy by the unimaginable physical and emotional stress of heart transplantation. That chapter alone should change the way we think about what we are doing in modern medicine, about doctors and patients.

One part of the book struck me as especially poignant. At the end, after the transplant, both he and his wife start having dreams in which they are accused of murder or some other heinous crime. Pensack analyzes these as guilt over the fact that his good fortune in receiving a heart transplant necessitated the death of a young healthy person. Heart transplantation, more than perhaps any other aspect of medicine, is a zero-sum game. For someone to win, someone has to lose.

It struck me that, in a sense, heart transplantation may be more emblematic than unique in this regard. Everything we do in medicine today embodies the same sort of contradiction. Our health care system is extravagant to the point of absurdity. We care for some individuals who are dying and who we know will die, and we treat their metastatic cancers, and their overwhelming fungal infections, their heart and lung and kidney and intestinal failure at enormous expense. At the same time, others go without prenatal care, mental health care, nursing home care, or treatment for drug addiction—the basic medical care that could save and transform their lives. In our crazy allocation system, it seems that some win and others lose and we can't explain why or how to avoid it.

International disparities are even more disturbing. In the United States we sometimes spend more on just a few patients than the entire health budgets of some countries. We spend money on growth hormone treatment to make short children taller, or antianxiety medication to relieve our existential angst, or sports medicine to improve our ability to enjoy skiing or golf, while millions of people in other countries die because their most basic health needs go unmet.

These stark and morally troubling contradictions seem inevitable, unavoidable, written into the system as if it were some giant lottery. A few years ago, twins were born in Chicago who were joined at the chest. Doctors there didn't want to operate, but other doctors in Philadelphia agreed to give it a try. One twin died, predictably, on the operating table. The other lived a year and then died. The story got a lot of press in Chicago. Reporters called to ask me, as an ethicist, whether I didn't think it was crazy to spend so much money on one child who had only a minuscule chance of survival while so many others were going without basic health services. In response, I quoted Samuel Shem, author of that modern medical classic *The House of God,* "That's not crazy, that's modern medicine." Our creation is extravagant, symbolic, irrational, and sometimes cruel, all in the name of a hopelessly idealistic standard that, as doctors, we should be uncompromisingly committed to the single patient in front of us. We don't want to be bureaucrats or bean counters.

In Pensack's account, thirty or forty doctors in ten medical centers around the country work together to discover and then apply new insights into the care of one patient. If you count the researchers who made it all possible, it would involve thousands. And yet, Pensack, though alive, is not healthy. He is sicker than ever. He needs a psychiatrist just to help him deal with the emotional trauma of what the medical care system has done to him. But you get the sense that he wouldn't have done it any differently. As disturbing as the book is, the writing of it is inevitably a sort of affirmation. Pensack is still alive. He has a voice.

Policy analysts talk about physician-induced demand for medical services. There are some medical interventions, they imply, that patients would never want or demand for themselves but that physicians nevertheless can successfully peddle, using their power, influence, and special knowledge. This phenomenon may explain part of the extraordinary growth of the health care industry over the past few decades but probably doesn't explain much. Most new health care innovations are not hard to sell. In many cases, demand is induced not by marketing gimmicks but by discovering treatments or cures that are neither self-serving nor unnecessary. We allow the blind to see. We stop the congenitally abnormal heart, correct its deformities, and restart it. We take half of a mother's liver from her body and give it to her child. As Paul Simon says, "These are the days of miracle and wonder. . . . Medicine is magical and magical is ordinary, the boy in the bubble, the baby with the baboon heart."[78] You don't have to induce demand for miracles.

But even the miraculous can become ordinary. One of the disturbing thing about the miracles of scientific discovery is how quickly we come to take them for granted. We're no longer in awe when a 747 takes off; we're grumpy because it is half an hour late. We're no longer in awe when we conceive a baby in a petri dish; we worry about whether insurance should pay for it. We're addicted to continuous surprise.

In Chicago, after Michael Jordan abruptly retired from basketball a few years ago, the fans had low expectations for the team. Then to everybody's surprise, the Bulls started winning without Michael. One sportswriter called it a *miraculous* season. Miraculous! That was the word he used. Then the team went into a slump. And what was the response? The fans started booing. They were no longer in awe of the miraculous; they'd come to expect it. When they booed Scottie Pippin, he snapped back that they never boo at the white guys. Tony Kukoc, a white guy from Croatia, wisely stayed out of the argument, perhaps out of a sense of the dangers of ethnic conflicts that surpassed even that of African Americans.

Is Scottie held to a higher standard? If so, is it because he is black? Such dilemmas seem to capture the public imagination to a greater degree than the dilemmas of resource allocation in health care. And they are not unrelated. Is there institutional racism among fans in the NBA? What is institutional racism? Is it possible for an institution to be immoral when every one of its members, individually, is moral?

There were not too many African Americans at the Society for Pediatric Research meetings. This was interesting because the meetings focused primarily on neonatal problems. One of the biggest neonatal problems in the United States today is the racial disparity in infant mortality. Black babies are twice as likely to die as white babies, and the disparity is increasing, in spite of all our miracles.[79] And yet, at the research meetings, it was mostly white folks staying in fancy hotels, talking about interleuken II, cytokines, and the Human Genome Project, as if the biochemical similarities between our patients were more important than the cultural, or racial, or economic differences.

People like to look back at other times or places and decry the moral backwardness of others. We want to see ourselves as having progressed, as standing at the pinnacle, as being better. How could other cultures have allowed slavery, or human sacrifice, and still imagine themselves moral, religious, admirable? Didn't it trouble people? Were they moral cretins? Future generations, looking back at us, will likely wonder how we could so comfortably have tolerated the inequality, cruelty, and injustice in our midst. How, they will ask, could we have allowed some citizens to live in rat-infested urban tenements while others basked by the pools of suburban country clubs? Didn't it trouble people? How could we have allowed sixth graders to obtain automatic weapons and take them to school? How could we have devoted so many resources to medical care for a few people with rare diseases and failed to provide prenatal care for pregnant women, immunizations or lead-free housing for our children? How could we tolerate the racial disparities? Didn't it bother people? they will ask. Why did we allocate resources to some endeavors but not to others?

Truth Telling and Opportunity Costs

Economists talk about opportunity costs, about how every dollar we spend on health care has to be thought of as a dollar that could be spent on something else, as an opportunity lost. They ask us to ask ourselves whether, if given the choice, we'd choose to spend a trillion dollars a year—that's four thousand dollars per year for every man, woman, and child in the country—on health care.

What, I wondered, would be the opportunity cost of telling the truth to our little nine-year-old with HIV? Her mother has already told her one thing. One cost of our telling would be that she would lose faith in her mother, that the abandonment she was facing by her mother's death and the fear she felt about her own would be compounded by a realization that her mother had deceived her. How can we put a value on that loss to measure it against the gains? What would the gains be?

The doctors might gain a sort of moral self-aggrandizement by telling the truth. This would be partly selfish. Their consciences would be eased. They would not have to suffer from participating in a deception or question whether the conventional moral wisdom was always correct. The hospital lawyers would be happy. Telling the truth is always good for risk management, although the fact that it is might make us question how much it really empowers patients.

Perhaps, and this is the most difficult argument, perhaps the child would gain something by being allowed to know and understand the truth about her own situation and to come to terms with it. Moral proponents of truth telling to children generally rely on this sort of hope, which, it turns out, is fairly utilitarian. That is, it rests on the belief that people will be better off knowing the truth. It doesn't accept, much less analyze, the possibility that in some situations people might not be able to handle so much truth, that truth can be emotionally devastating.

Many people, hearing this case, conclude that the child must have known that she had AIDS. After all, she was in a teaching hospital. Tongues must have slipped. She was not a helpless infant. She had ways of piecing things together. What if we assume that she did know? What then might be gained by telling her?

Here, proponents of truth telling usually imagine a scenario of coming to terms with the truth, the gratifying emotional release that might follow a tearful acknowledgment, the freeing up of psychic energy that might be redirected from deception to love. This, it seems to me, is a comically simplistic view of human psychic life. Coming to terms with truth is rarely so easy.

It seems psychologically plausible to me that she does know but also knows, as prescient nine-year-olds might, that her mom and grandma have chosen their own way of dealing with it. Perhaps she understands, intuitively, their vulnerability; perhaps she's protecting them; perhaps denial represents a sort of incantation against the truth, a source of hope, solidarity, maybe even power. These ideas may seem far-fetched but, to me, they seem no less plausible that the formulaic belief that the truth will set us free.

What about the grandma? She was already losing a daughter and a granddaughter to a cruel and brutal death. She had failed to protect her daughter and granddaughter from the new and almost unimaginable scourge of AIDS. She had nothing at all to offer them after her lifetime of experience and sacrifice but stories, fictions, beautiful lies. Take that away and she would lose the sense that she at least had a role to play in telling the stories that would shape the deaths of those she loved. Who knows what secret meanings AIDS had for her or her daughter or her granddaughter? Who knew how they were thinking about death? As the story was told and as such stories often play out, nobody knew and nobody really cared. They were characters in our morality tale, already typecast as villains.

Our health care system today is a strange morality tale indeed. The contradictions of the medical enterprise are straining society to the breaking point. The Clintons' attempt to forthrightly address the issue of health care reform failed under a barrage of misinformation and lies from various interests too vested even to identify themselves by name. The health reform task force was accused of being "secretive," even though the details of its plans were in the *Times* and *Wall Street Journal* every day. Current efforts at health reform are shielded from public scrutiny in a way that the "secret" task force meetings never were. Key policy decisions are now corporate secrets or are carefully veiled in the uninterpretable language of the bureaucrats. Health care is very much in the news, but it's hard to tell who will pay for what for whom and when and why. And that seems to be the way we like it. We can't even begin to discuss honestly how resources are allocated, who gets what, and who should. Subterfuge and dissembling are at the core. In health reform, as in other places, the conventional wisdom seems to be that if, politically, you can't say anything nice, don't say anything at all. Perhaps one of the reasons that we want to tell the truth to children is to salvage some sense of ourselves as honest people in a world where all the evidence suggests otherwise.

One problem with doctors and truth telling is that we're not very good storytellers. We cannot imagine medical scenarios as real tragedies or our patients as tragic heroes. We cannot imagine ourselves as shamans or healers. We seem to be having trouble remembering what it means to be a doctor, or seeing the connections between what we call morality and risk management, between the narrow view of truth telling that turns doctors into providers and patients into clients and the larger problems in medicine today. There is nothing profound at the core any more. We thrive on the mundane. We want to reduce the doctor-patient relationship to a contract, the disease to an abnormal blood test. We imagine that moral rules can be powerful enough to transform tragedy into something simple and noble. But they can't. AIDS is a disease that kills the young and the healthy in the prime of their lives, a disease that a mother can give to her child and from which both can die together, a disease that largely exempts the old, so that grandmothers must watch the deaths of their progeny. Perhaps, in the case of the nine-year-old, the grandmother was unwilling to admit even to herself that death was inevitable or to think about what might follow. Perhaps she was wondering about who would take care of her once she no longer had people she should or would care for. Perhaps what she was expressing was not falsehood but faith, not a moral lapse but a different conception of morality that was bigger and richer than ours.

Truth telling is important, but it was the last thing these people needed. They needed someone to listen to them rather than talk to them. They didn't need facts, they needed compassion, concern, caring. This was not the time to talk about rights or to make moral judgments. This was a situation in which ordinary notions of morality were being sucked into a black hole of tragedy, where the task was to help a family create a myth strong enough and strange enough and rhythmic enough to comfort them at a time when all the ordinary myths were inadequate. It was a time for heroes, not actuaries.

Locating Ethics

We had another case recently that continues to haunt and trouble me. The patient was a seventeen-year-old girl from an Orthodox Jewish community on the East Coast. Three weeks prior to admission, she had gone to her rabbi's wife to discuss Jewish laws regarding marriage in preparation for her upcoming wedding. As was the custom in her community, the wedding had been arranged. She had met her fiancé only once.

In the course of the marital counseling, it was discovered that she had dysfunctional uterine bleeding. This led to a medical evaluation, the eventual discovery of uterine cancer, and referral to our hospital, one of the top centers in the world for treatment of this cancer. The recommended treatment was radiation followed by a hysterectomy, which would of course leave her infertile.

When her father heard the medical recommendations, he requested of the doctors that they not tell his daughter that the treatment would leave her infertile. He thought that that news would be emotionally devastating—both in itself and because he feared that it might lead to the cancellation of her marriage. Because she would be infertile, her fiancé would no longer be obligated to marry her. The call for the ethics consult asked, "Do we have to tell her that she will be infertile?"

Well, in one sense, it was easy. Informed consent, respect for persons, truth telling. From a risk-management point of view, it was a no-brainer. You tell her; if she refuses treatment, that's her choice. It may be tragic, but it isn't a tort. Treat without consent and she sues later; it is at least malpractice and maybe assault and battery. From a bioethics perspective, these legal considerations reflected appropriate moral concerns.

Not to tell would be paternalistic, and in bioethics there is no greater sin than paternalism, although that might be hard to explain to her father.

But from another perspective, it seemed a little more complex. Were we really concerned about the patient's interest or about the hospital's? Whenever ethics and risk management agree, a red flag should go up. Furthermore, the legal and moral principles that we were relying on were neither timeless nor universal. If she had not been in the United States, or if it had been twenty-five years earlier, nobody would have told her. She was a minor. Her parents had the right to make decisions for her. In addition, her religion did not acknowledge the importance of autonomy. As her father said, "She must have the treatment. It is required by law. Why add to her suffering now, when she needs hope and strength?" Clearly, he had her best interests at heart.

The ethics committee meeting was a little acrimonious and inconclusive.[80] Arguments flew about beneficence and autonomy, patriarchal religions and sexism, culture, families and parents. The conversation was intense.

"She has to be told that she will be infertile. Her consent would not be informed consent without that information. You'd be sterilizing someone without her permission."

"Well, strictly speaking, *we* wouldn't be sterilizing her. Her tumor is making her sterile. Without treatment, it would continue to grow, and she would not only be sterile but would die. With treatment, she would also be sterile, but she might live."

"She feels that her life wouldn't be worth living if she is sterile."

"We don't know what she feels, just what her father thinks she will feel."

"We don't want to know what she feels."

"How can a seventeen-year-old make a decision like this?"

"What does the law say?"

"Whose law, ours or hers?"

"It shouldn't depend on the law; it's a moral issue. What's right is right, no matter what the law says."

"Tell that to the judge."

"Tell it to the rabbi!"

"It wouldn't be right to treat a seventeen-year-old without consent if she can understand the treatment and the alternatives. It is wrong to sterilize anybody, no matter what age, without telling them what you are doing."

"She's already sterile."

"Maybe."

"Definitely."

"It would be even more definite after a hysterectomy."

"We're only considering not telling because she is a girl. If this was a case of a boy with a seminoma who required castration, we would certainly tell him, and let him decide. We just think that a man without balls may not have a life worth living, but a girl without ovaries does."

"Is that discriminatory against women? Or against men?"

"Could she donate eggs?"

"No, she would have to be pretreated to stimulate follicle development. That would take time, and the hormones might stimulate the growth of her tumor and make her prognosis worse."

"Given that she is already infertile, what difference does it make if we tell her now or after treatment has begun?"

"The difference is whether we are respecting her autonomy."

"But her culture doesn't respect autonomy."

"It should!"

"Oh, that's great. Informed consent as a form of philosophic fascism. Why are we so intolerant of other systems of belief?"

"We're intolerant of lying."

"It wouldn't be lying to tell her we're doing what we think is best to cure her disease."

"She'd never trust doctors again."

"But she'd be alive to distrust them."

We gave the gynecology service lots of good arguments on both sides but no consensus. They decided that she had to be told.

A family meeting was convened. The family was quite uncomfortable by the idea of this meeting, but they did their best and asked lots of questions. The gynecologist answered them all:

"Is there no other treatment?"

"None."

"Could she donate eggs for IVF later? A surrogate mother?"

"No, it would take too long and the hormonal stimulation might stimulate the tumor."

"If she had radiation but not surgery, mightn't she conceive?"

"No. The radiation will destroy her ovaries."

"Someday, maybe, a uterus transplant?"

"Impossible."

The doctor didn't pull any punches. He wanted to tell her the honest truth, to make certain she understood, not to give any false hopes. He succeeded. After an hour of such talk, the conversation ebbed to silence. A pall hung over the room. Finally, the girl muttered something and walked out of the room. Her mother ran after her. Her father slumped down in his chair. "What'd she say?" we asked. "She said she doesn't want the treatment." He looked at us as if we were monsters.

Did we do the right thing? We followed all the rules. Our actions were based on adherence to the most idealistic moral principles. In a certain sense, what we did was unassailable. In the most difficult and trying circumstances, we had confronted ugly truths instead of hiding from them. We had helped a patient, who clearly had the capacity to make her own decisions, to understand the choices before her, and to make a choice based on her own deeply felt personal moral values. This was a triumph for patient autonomy, for feminism, for children's rights, a culmination of twenty-five years of work in health law, civil liberties, and bioethics. But it felt as if we had betrayed everything that medicine stands for and had become zealots in a cause that looked less like moral excellence and more like political dogma.

Unlike many stories, this one had a happy ending. The girl returned a few days after the family conference saying she'd changed her mind and wanted treatment. She signed the consent form without reading it. What had changed? Over the weekend, she'd spoken to her rabbi. Without any disrespect for the doctors, he said, "If God wants you to have children, you'll have children. Not to believe that would be worse than death. It would be idolatry."

Her fiancé did not forsake her. In fact, as we were later to learn, he spent two hours each day praying for her, reciting the entire Book of Psalms every morning. Six months later, her cancer in remission, they were married. They planned to adopt children.

A happy ending! So what's the problem? As Abraham Lincoln noted in describing the start of the Civil War, everybody struggled to do what was right as they saw the right. The rabbi interpreted Torah and Talmud to come to a truth that differed somewhat from the truth of the doctors. Could the doctors have offered hope in the same way the rabbi did? Perhaps. But they felt morally bound to convey the truths of science, not religion. The parents stood with a foot in each truth community, clearly trusting the doctors with their daughter's life but not trusting the doctors' moral vision. The young woman chose life over death and obedience to her parents and teachers over an individualistic tragedy that her doctors and lawyers would have allowed.

What about the fiancé? He, it seems to me, went beyond what was required or expected. How many teenage boys would remain steadfastly loyal to a girl they had met only once, and marry someone whom they knew would never be able to have a baby, might even have trouble having sex, and might die? Caught up in a situation beyond his experience or imagination, he made a choice that embodied the highest moral ideals and that determined the ultimate outcome of the story. The happy ending came about, it seems to me, not because we necessarily did the right thing but because he did. The happy ending was not a triumph for individualism, autonomy, patients' rights, or truth telling. It was a triumph for steadfastness, loyalty, interdependence, and faith. It was less about people following the rules and more about people living in a world in which situations constantly force them to go beyond the rules. The ethics committee, it seemed to me, was doing something that had far less to do with ethics than what that young man was doing. And what he did, rather than what they did, is what really mattered.

Archeologists recently uncovered a skeleton that they believe may be the oldest human being ever discovered. Four-and-a-half million years old. Debates turned on issues of morphology and whether the bone structure was such that we could say this was or was not really a human being. Humans may go back that far, and even then they would have been newcomers on the geologic scene. But for me, the evidence of humanity always has less to do with morphology and more to do culture. Humans live in communities. We bury our dead. We care for one another, even once the breath of life is gone. This, more than cranial size or tooth structure, or the ability to transplant livers or sequence the genome, makes us unique. It is to these qualities that we will need to turn for the moral wisdom to guide us through the next few years or decades in medicine.

Aristotle excelled as both a scientist and a moralist. His biologic investigations were state of the art for centuries. But today, we read his ethics with a sense of urgency for what it can teach us about how we should live, and we read his science for what it tells us about his ethics. Whatever moral knowledge may be, it is not cumulative in the way that science is cumulative. We do not take Aristotle's ethics and build on it, the way we can take Newton's science and build on it. Hence, we don't make progress in ethics in quite the same way we make progress in science. Instead of a sense of progress, ethics seems to have a frustrating circularity about it. We go round and round the same issues.

But it is not really circular, even though it is not really linear either. It is a different kind of knowledge. It is knowledge that is not outside us but must be welded to our souls over and over again: each child must learn the same lessons, each doctor experience it personally. Nobody can mass produce it. We can teach doctors about do-not-resuscitate orders, or informed consent, or euthanasia until we're blue in the face and people will be no more ethical. They will learn only how to follow the rules. But to care for a dying patient, to allow the enormousness and mystery and inevitability of death wash over us, to respond to it with all the anger and compassion and helplessness that has always characterized our responses to death, and to hang in there, to continue to pray and not run away, to be there for another human being, that is another matter.

Nobody can discover it for us so we won't have to discover it ourselves, nobody can teach us how to do it so that we can memorize it and go on to the next lesson. Instead, all we can do is celebrate in poetry and song those who have learned the lessons and whose lives exemplify moral truths. And we can hope that their examples inspire us to comparable courage when our time comes. Such virtues must be learned over and over again, by every individual, in every generation.

In his last novel, *The Thanatos Syndrome*, physician Walker Percy imagines surreptitious researchers lacing the water supply of a few Louisiana parishes with a drug that makes people happier, less prone to violent crime, and better bridge players.[81] The drug eliminates all feelings of guilt or anxiety. It also decreases sexual inhibitions and unfortunately leads to a small outbreak of child sexual abuse. Percy accuses both modern philosophy and modern medicine of misguidedly trying to do what the drug does: cure us of guilt, anxiety, or suffering and at the same time "cure" us of the possibility of morality. Discontent seems to be the price of civilization. Near the end, one of the renegade researchers is discussing events with a psychiatrist who blew the whistle on him: "We were after the same thing," he says. "The greatest good, the highest quality of life for the greatest number. In the end there is no reason to allow a single child to suffer needlessly, a single old person to linger in pain" (p. 376). But the hero disagrees. He is groping toward the view that there is something more important than curing disease or relieving suffering, that perhaps even suffering and disease can be holy or beneficial. Percy asks us to think about the goals and to wonder together about the price that we might be willing to pay for lives without pain and deaths with dignity.

William Carlos Williams, a pediatrician and poet, knew better than most that, in the end, the doctor's task must be assessed by something other than mortality statistics or other conventional measures of success. Cost-benefit analyses can identify but cannot solve moral dilemmas, because, in the end, we each have to define the terms that are represented by the variables in the equation. We need to figure out what is a cost and what is a benefit. Williams has an almost stoical acceptance of suffering when he writes, "We know the plane will crash, the train will be derailed. And we know why. No one cares, no one can care. We get the news and discount it, and we are quite right in doing so. It is trivial. But the haunted news I get from some obscure patient's eyes is not trivial. It is profound: whole academies of learning, whole ecclesiastical hierarchies are founded upon it."[82]

For Williams, the mysteries of science are dwarfed by the mysterious process by which he, as a physician, becomes drawn in by his patients. He is not interested in impossible systems that promise the relief of human suffering. Instead, he is interested in the human capacity to respond to the claims that other individuals make upon us with a look, a sigh, or a sob.

Medicine today is facing many problems, many changes. Doctors fifty years from now will do things that we cannot imagine, just as we do things that our forebears would have found miraculous. There may not even be doctors as we know them today. And yet, doctors today do some of the same things that doctors have always done and will always do. That permanence, it seems to me, has nothing to do with science, nothing to do with technology, nothing to do with whether we work in fee-for-service solo practices, HMOs, the British National Health Service, or the Veterans Administration. It doesn't have much to do with tort reform, managed care, or "safe havens" from conflict-of-interest legislation. And, oddly enough, it doesn't even have much to do with whether what we do works or doesn't work. Instead, it has to do with whether, like William Carlos Williams, we nurture the capacity to respond to "the haunted news" we get from "some obscure patient's eyes." No matter how good our science gets or how our health system is organized, someone will always have to do that.

In some ways, the question is not whether we should tell the truth but whether we are going to conceptualize the doctor-patient interaction as something legalistic, commercial, and contractual or as something religous, spiritual, or artistic. Each interaction would demand a different sort of truth. Our patients ought to get the truth, but we should not fall into the trap of thinking there is just one truth. Dietrich Bonhoffer's *Ethics,* written while he was in prison awaiting execution for his part in a conspiracy to assassinate Adolf Hitler, has a section on truth telling.

There, he writes, "The cynic who claims 'to speak the truth' at all times and in all places to all men in the same way, displays nothing but a lifeless image of the truth. . . . He wounds shame, desecrates mystery, breaks confidence, betrays the community in which he lives, and laughs arrogantly at the devastation he has wrought and at the human weakness which 'cannot bear the truth.'"[83] Bonhoffer had it just right. None of us can bear too much truth, least of all doctors. Even in our desire to tell the truth, it seems, we're kidding ourselves.

So I, at least, am convinced that certain forms of truth are overrated. I don't think the little girl would be better off getting her parenteral nutrition, dialysis, and mechanical ventilation while she withers away in a state-of-the-art ICU, where in all probability her pain and suffering will be inadequately treated while every measurable physiologic parameter is carefully charted every eight hours, and knowing that she has a disease we call AIDS. Or if, by contrast, she would be better off lying on a bed of flowers wrapped in blankets while everyone in her village danced around her and smoked peyote. We may not be able to offer her the flowers and peyote, but we might at least let her grandmother read her fairy tales about good witches, gods and spirits, or worlds where girls never get sick, or never grow up, and tell her how she'll go to bed and sleep peacefully and wake up cured in a beautiful countryside where her mother will be healthy and happy and they'll all play together.

Most children in the world who die don't get dialysis, parenteral nutrition, or the truth. Might not two out of three be enough?

I can't imagine how I would behave if my daughter and granddaughter were dying of AIDS, whether I would choose the brutal truth or a comforting lie. But I do know that, whatever I chose, I would not want a doctor judging the morality of my decision. I would want a doctor who could listen to me, comfort me, hug me, cry with me, or just be with me, but not one who would judge me. Sometimes, perhaps, even in the United States, the best medicine might still be a comforting lie.

7

On Mistakes and Truth Telling

I've made quite a few mistakes in my time. They come back to haunt me
late at night. Missing a diagnosis, prescribing the wrong drug, botching a
procedure. Sometimes, patients have died as a result of my mistakes.
Other times, my mistakes have increased their suffering. When they
come back to me, late at night, I hold court in my mind, replaying events,
wondering whether they were honest mistakes, forgivable mistakes, or if
not, how I can go on. Some of the worst were when I was a resident.

My third year as a pediatrics resident, I was cross-covering the neonatal intensive care unit (NICU). I was working all day in the genetics
clinic, then covering the neonatal unit from 5:00 P.M. until 8:00 A.M.,
then going back to the genetics clinic for another day.

I had recently gotten married, and my wife was pregnant, so the genetics
clinic was a disturbing place. Each patient was another page in the huge
catalogue of things that could go wrong. It was the ultimate random-num-
ber machine. The clinical geneticist tried to recognize each constellation of
abnormalities and to match the child to a list of syndromes. The syndromes
were generally named after the doctors who first described them, so that in
a day we would see Downs, Williams, Smith-Lemli-Opitz, Rubenstein-
Taybi, or Russel-Silver, each an amalgam of malformation, dysfunctions,
anomalies. It seemed as if God did play dice with the universe.

From there, I'd go to the NICU. It was 1983, the end of a decade of
phenomenal, unprecedented progress in neonatal care. Mortality rates

for premature babies had dropped from 80 percent to 20 percent. The atmosphere was heady, exultant. Neonatologists were the Green Berets of pediatrics: daring, elitist, a breed apart. They not only saved lives, making themselves heroes within the specialty, but also kept hospital beds full, making them the heroes of the hospital administrators. Miraculous cures in neonatal care took months, required a lot of technology, and led to the creation of a whole new subspecialty that quickly became the largest subspecialty in pediatrics.

I hated it. The first time I walked into the NICU, I nearly passed out. The blood drained from my head, my heart began to race, a wave of nausea passed over me. I broke out in a sweat and went to sit down. The babies were disconcertingly insubstantial against the machines to which they were attached. Ventilators. Monitors. Intravenous pumps with three or four separate solutions running at once. Some of the babies were swaddled in plastic wrap, others seemed to be baking under the severe glow of the phototherapy lights. There was a steady hum and beep. Everybody who worked there was female, and there was something insectlike about their quiet purposefulness. Nobody seemed to be a mother to any of these babies. I wondered if perhaps they'd just hatched.

The night I was cross-covering, I got the sign-out from one of my fellow residents. Forty babies, some critically ill, some stable. Most of them had the same problems, all associated with prematurity: lung disease, bleeding into their immature brains, bowel necrosis, infections, seizures. We knew the drill. Three years ago, I'd almost passed out. Now, I felt like I could do it in my sleep. I was wrong.

By midnight, I'd made my rounds, had a snack, admitted two new babies, and crept off to the call room for a fitful nap. I was so exhausted that sometimes I could actually drift off for a few minutes between pages. Preemies filled my dreams, umbilical catheters snaking out of their little belly-buttons and wrapping around my neck. The babies and their intravenous lines writhed and twisted together, dancing together toward survival or death. The dreams were partly morbid, partly sensual, partly mocking.

Beep. Beep. Beep.

One of the more stable babies in the "back room" had a rapid heart rate. I went to look. His monitor was shrieking. Three hundred beats per minute. His perfusion was OK. He was sweating a little, a sign of distress. I looked at the sign-out sheet. "Three month old, congential heart disease. Has had two open heart operations. Episodes of supraventricular tachycardia. Try ice. Try Verapamil. Call Cardiology."

Even now, I don't like to think about what happened next. I still haven't come to grips with my own behavior, my own mistake. I play it over and over again in my head and, in the replay, it comes out different. I call Cardiology. The ice works.

Ice. An unusual treatment. Here's what is supposed to happen. Sometimes, the electrical control system of the heart doesn't work. The heart can start to race. If you dunk the baby's face in ice water, it can stimulate a reflex that causes the heart rate to slow down. I tried it. It didn't work. I tried it again. It still didn't work. Verapamil was a new drug, just licensed, that was supposed to be effective. However, some case reports that had just come out reported that, in newborns, it sometimes caused cardiac arrests. I hadn't read those case reports. I hadn't read much. I probably should have. Two years before, Verapamil hadn't been available. Two years later, everybody knew that it shouldn't be used in neonates. But that year, at two in the morning, I gave a baby a dose. The baby's heart stopped. Like that. Three hundred to zero in the blink of an eye.

Holy shit.

Start CPR. Intubate. Epi. Calcium. Chest compressions. We squeezed his little chest. And squeezed. And squeezed.

Did I make a mistake? I'm still not sure. I did what I was told to do, something that seemed right at the time but turned out horribly wrong. There were, perhaps, things I could have known, things I should have known. I should have called to ask for help. I could have tried the ice again. I could have done anything but what I did.

I've made other mistakes. Missed diagnoses. Botched procedures. Said stupid or offensive things to patients. I've failed to return phone calls, not checked lab results in time, misread X-rays. When I wake at night thinking of them, I wonder when the lawsuit will come. I imagine myself pleading guilty.

Sometimes, I review other cases for lawsuits. Doctors make a lot of mistakes. There are a lot of bad outcomes. Some patients die, others are permanently injured. When the cases are scrutinized, in retrospect, there are always problems. Things seldom go perfectly. The records of events are always incomplete, sketchy. The stories of what happened can be reconstructed and retold and reinterpreted in many ways.

Narrative Reconstruction and Moral Evasion

At the University of Chicago, we have an ethics consultation service. We get called about a couple of cases a week. Most have to do with patients who are dying, decisions about how their lives should end. The patient is incompetent and has no living will or durable power of attorney. The family members cannot agree about what should be done, or the medical consultants disagree about the prognosis. Our role, as consultants in such cases, is generally somewhere between arbitration, conflict resolution, and psychotherapy. Seldom is there fundamental disagreement about what is morally permissible, although there may be disagreement about what is morally preferable. The relative ease with which we generally achieve consensus in these cases is evidence of one of the major societal successes of bioethics. Since the 1970s, when doctors and lawyers both argued that it would be homicide to take Karen Quinlan off her ventilator, we have changed the way we think about death and dying and come to grips with the awesome new responsibilities our phenomenal medical technology creates.

But there are other cases where no such consensus has developed, and where the fundamental issues seem deeper and closer to questions about what it means to be a doctor. Generally, these issues involve cases in which doctors have special access to knowledge, and claim special privileges. One of the most controversial of these has been when doctors claim a special privilege to withhold the truth.

There are many ways to evade the truth. Doctors may not want to disclose a patient's dismal diagnosis if the diagnosis is severe. This is generally justified as a way of preserving the patient's hope or good spirits. Don't tell him that he has terminal, metastatic cancer. This lie goes back at least to Hippocrates, and was best portrayed, and criticized, by

Tolstoy. In *The Death of Ivan Illych,* Tolstoy writes, "What tormented Ivan Illych most was the deception, which for some reason they all accepted, that he was not dying but was simply ill. . . . That deception tortured him—their not wishing to admit what they all knew and what he knew, but wanting to lie to him concerning his terrible disposition, and wishing and forcing him to participate in that lie."[84] Long before modern bioethics even had a name, Tolstoy recognized the degradation inherent in this approach. It has few defenders today.

Without actually lying, however, doctors may withhold prognostic information or shade the truth about a patient's actual circumstances. This is somewhat easier to justify than an outright lie because prognosis is a much more iffy business than diagnosis. Even in Tolstoy, the specialist gives a guarded prognosis. "In reply to the timid question Ivan Illych, with eyes glistening with fear and hope, put to him as to whether there was a chance for recovery, [the specialist] said that he could not vouch for it but there was a possibility" (p. 585). There is always a possibility!

The impulse to soften the blow is irresistible, born of empathy and concern. It is not something doctors do as doctors. It is something doctors do as caring people. In Philip Roth's memoir about caring for his father during a terminal illness, Roth finds himself doing the same thing.[85] The doctor tells Philip that his father, Herman Roth, has "a massive brain tumor." Philip can't tell this to his dad. His first impulse is to lie. He tells him that the MRI showed nothing. Then, when he realizes that he can't get away with that, he tells part of the truth. He recounts his own evasions:

> "You have a serious problem," I began, "but it can be dealt with. You have a tumor in your head. Dr. Myerson says that given the location, the chances are 95% that it is benign." I had intended, like Myerson, to be candid and describe it as large, but I couldn't. That there was a tumor seemed enough for him to take. . . . "It's pressing on the facial nerve. That's what caused the paralysis." Myerson had told me that it was wrapped around the facial nerve, but I couldn't say that either. (p. 66)

For a doctor, as for a son, a more rigorous standard of truth telling would call for a certain heartlessness.

A third type of problem with truth telling occurs when doctors make mistakes. Should patients be informed when the doctor errs? This has received a lot less attention than the other two types but probably comes up much more often. We recently were consulted about the following case:

> A thirty-eight-year-old married woman with two children developed breast cancer. Conventional treatment failed, and she elected to undergo intensive chemotherapy and bone marrow transplantation. She was informed, and understood, that her chances for survival were low, probably less than 20 percent. After the bone marrow transplant she had a stormy course. She developed severe graft-versus-host disease, renal failure, and multiple infections. She never left the ICU. Two weeks after the transplant, she developed sepsis and had a cardiorespiratory arrest. CPR was unsuccessful and the patient died.
>
> A few days later, during a routine postmortem review, it was discovered that the intravenous fluids that were provided during the resuscitation contained ten times the normal dose of potassium chloride. This increased dose could have killed a healthy person, and may have contributed to this woman's death. The doctor asked the ethicists whether he should tell the family about the mistake.

We argued vigorously. One question was whether the mistake *caused* the woman's death. It was unclear. It would have been better, of course, to have given her the proper dose of potassium chloride. However, even with the proper dose, her chances for survival were extremely low. The mistake may have been a small, incremental, addition to the sepsis, renal failure, cancer, and graft-versus-host disease. It may have *contributed* to her death. On the other hand, she was clearly dying at the time it occurred. She might have been dead already by the time the inappropriate fluids were administered.

Still, some said, the family has the right to know. After all, we know. We have an obligation to tell them what we know and what it means. They should, of course, be told of our uncertainty about the relevance of the clinical information and of the likelihood of her death even without the error. In other words, they should know everything we know.

Others argued that the information was meaningless and irrelevant, and that it may even be harmful. The family was dealing with enough tragedy, they said. To give them this ambiguous and questionably useful information would only add confusion, anger, guilt, and suffering. It may interrupt their mourning process by creating a diversion.

But, others replied, not to tell them looks like a cover-up. If they find out someday, they'll be much more upset, and will be more likely to sue us. If we tell them, we'll have done the right thing legally.

Yes, came the reply, but if we tell them, it will be an invitation to sue. They probably won't find out, and won't sue, unless we tell them. We turned to the lawyers, who shrugged and said that whatever we did, we should be sure to document it well. Truth telling is best, someone said. Not always, another replied. We ended up a hung jury, and told the attending that either option was acceptable. He didn't tell the family.

Recently, a discussion on a bioethics forum on the Internet replayed this debate. It was a general discussion, with many different cases batted around. Someone had injected a knee with estrogen instead of cortisone; someone had caused a respiratory arrest by giving a patient too much morphine; someone missed a crucial diagnosis. Did they have an obligation to tell?

Interestingly, both in our local ethics committee and in cyberspace, the lawyers and philosophers argued for a rigorous standard of truth telling, and the physicians hemmed and hawed, not quite knowing what counterarguments they could make but somehow feeling that something less than total disclosure was acceptable. So here is the question: Did these evasive, hemming-and-hawing doctors have a moral leg to stand on or were they just doing a little professional emotional self-protection and damage control?

Silent Worlds

There are only a few works in the medical ethics canon that deal in any depth with mistakes or with truth telling. In *The Silent World of Doctor and Patient*, Jay Katz makes an impassioned and compelling case for more honest communication between doctors and patients.[86] He argues that doctors emotionally abandon patients precisely at the moments when patients need them the most, that is, when the patients face heart-wrenching and psychically draining choices among difficult therapeutic options or when patients are dying. Katz theorizes that it is the doctors' own psychic conflicts and tensions that lead them at these moments to abandon patients to a dreadful silence. In Katz's view, the tendency to soften the blow and shade the truth is not compassion but a sort of emotional cowardice, protecting not the patients but the doctors.

Communication about mistakes seems to be a closely related communication issue, but it doesn't come up in Katz's book. Mistakes are not even mentioned in the index. In the otherwise fairly quiet world of doctor and patient, the silence surrounding this issue is particularly profound.

Charles Bosk wrote about the way surgical training programs deal with errors among trainees. His *Forgive and Remember* describes in great detail a variety of customs and practices for dealing with error: various types of sanctions and corrections, various classifications of errors. The program he studies is a pyramid program. There are more first-year residents than fifth-year residents, and Bosk analyzes the decisions of attendings to keep residents or let them go, the factors they consider in judging quality. They notice and evaluate all sorts of errors, and make fine distinctions among them. He describes the ritual of the surgical "morbidity and mortality conferences," in which senior surgeons confess their own errors, and are criticized by their colleagues. Puzzled at first, Bosk eventually realizes that this ritualistic confession of mistakes among colleagues is a way of acknowledging error without disclosing it outside the profession, and thus of solidifying and reinforcing the power of the senior attendings, who are seen as strong enough to confess their errors to their colleagues.[87]

Again, however, as in Katz's book, there is no mention or discussion of communicating errors to patients. Further, although Bosk was an ethnographer studying how doctors deal with error, there are no episodes in which he observes anybody telling patients about errors. The doctors seem to assume that the patients don't know.

Doctors who are not in training seldom tell patients or their colleagues about mistakes. J. F. Christensen and colleagues interviewed family practitioners and found that most remembered mistakes, but few had talked about their mistakes to colleagues, family, or friends.[88] The interviewers didn't even ask about disclosure to patients.

There is some evidence that patients do know about their doctors' mistakes. Many books by patients contain accounts of errors by physicians. In Roth's book, he describes how the diagnosis of a brain tumor was missed by a number of physicians.[89] Arthur Frank wrote about his own bout with cancer, and he also recounts a series of misdiagnoses and the complications that resulted from giving him the wrong drug or the wrong dose.[90] Oliver Sacks, a physician, wrote a memoir about a severe leg injury he sustained while mountain climbing and the treatment he received for it.[91] He tells in gory detail of the failure of his surgeon to diagnose a severe denervation injury that Sacks himself tried in vain to describe to him. Robert Pensack, another physician-patient, relates how he was nearly killed by a cardiothoracic surgeon who hadn't read the instructions for a new type of pacemaker that he had just inserted.[92] In almost no books do doctors or patients discuss a process by which such mistakes are or should or could be disclosed. It is as if there is no expectation on either side that the mistakes will be disclosed.

David Hilfiker is one of the few doctors who has broken the silence and taboo on the disclosure issue. In his disturbing 1984 essay "Facing Our Mistakes," in the *New England Journal of Medicine,* and in his memoir of life as a family practitioner in rural Minnesota, which he titled *Healing the Wounds,* Hilfiker catalogues the sorts of mistakes he made during his years in practice: misreading an X-ray, not adequately assessing the emergent nature of a patient's complaints, taking too long to get an IV into a newborn to give glucose, mistakenly aborting a fetus that he thought had died. His cases range from diagnostic judgments to technical lapses to inexcusable errors.[93] Reading his list as a doctor, I could remember making some of those mistakes, imagine making some, and dread making others. And I wasn't the only one. Letters poured into the journal. "Who among us," wrote James Sarfeh, "cannot describe similar personal 'horror stories' which through the years become firmly encased skeletons in the closets of our minds." "We should learn from our mistakes, not be crucified for them," wrote David Gregory. Interestingly, a nonphysician, Ellen Ingber, wrote that from a patient's perspective,

Hilfiker's confession leaves her sympathetic but uneasy. She wants to believe in perfect physicians as "a last bastion of security."[94]

Hilfiker reasons that telling patients of our mistakes is good because the burdens of physicianhood are too heavy; we should tell for the good of our souls. His rationale is that we physicians need forgiveness for our mistakes in order to maintain spiritual health, and this forgiveness can come only from patients. In some sense, this proposal puts a burden on patients to care for their physicians.

One of the surprising things about Hilfiker's essay is that, for all its blunt candor and shocking self-revelation, it was essentially an isolated event. I did a literature search of the five years prior to his essay and of the years since. There are only a few other articles that address mistakes or errors and truth telling or disclosure. Ely and colleagues interviewed fifty-three family physicians about mistakes that they had made.[95] Many of the mistakes had resulted in patients' deaths. The study tried to find the more common perceived causes of the mistakes in order to prevent future mistakes. There was no discussion about communicating mistakes to patients. Some of the articles approach the issue from the legal perspective, and talk about patients' right to information or recount lawsuits based on the right, but such suits are rare. More recent articles about mistakes in medicine are written from the perspective of quality assurance. They are seen as system problems rather than individual problems, and the proposed solutions are in the management and design of systems to help avoid errors. Again, the writers generally don't delve into the issue of disclosure to patients.

Definitional Problems

One problem is that it is difficult to decide what is or is not an error. Like many things that are undefinable without being indeterminate, there is a spectrum of events that are clearly recognizable as errors. There is another spectrum of events that have bad outcomes. However, the two categories are not always related. Some errors lead to no bad outcomes. Some have only minimal consequences. The doctor who substituted estrogen for cortisone when he injected a patient's knee discovered his mistake and immediately called his patient. The patient said his knee felt much better. This was certainly an error. However, it may have been beneficial for the patient. Giving twice the dose of an antibiotic is clearly an error but generally one without consequences.

Similarly (or perhaps contrapuntally), there are many bad outcomes that cannot be traced to particular errors: endotracheal tubes fall out, transfusions cause bad reactions, surgery patients develop postoperative infections. In many cases, we can think about possible causes and even assign some sort of probabilistic association but cannot definitely pin down any particular action as an error.

Lori Andrews and her colleagues tried to study errors in the intensive care units at our hospital. The study was motivated by events that occurred when the chief of surgery was hospitalized in the medical ICU with chest pain. He noticed many errors in his care, some potentially life-threatening. He bravely speculated that there would be fewer errors in the surgical intensive care unit and invited us to study it.

It took a while to come up with a workable definition of an error. The authors ended up being unable to classify events precisely as errors and, instead, developed the notion of events about which people raised questions, or what they called "eyebrow-raising events." This included situations where medicines were given late, or X-rays were misread, or dressings were not changed appropriately, or drugs were given to patients who had indicated that they were allergic to them. Many such events were found. Most had no adverse consequences or minor adverse consequences. Many were promptly discovered and corrected. Others were discovered much later. By this methodology, they would not have found errors that had not been discovered at all. (If an error occurs and nobody discovers it, is it really an error? If a tree falls in the forest . . .) Most discussion of and response to "eyebrow-raising events" were confined within the health care team.[96]

Charles Bosk eventually developed a classification scheme for errors which, although imprecise, captures something of the topography of this difficult terrain. Some errors, he states, are clearly "technical." In surgical training, they are generally errors of operative technique. An artery is nicked, a knot tied too loosely. Such errors are seen as inevitable and as morally neutral, as long as they are recognized promptly and dealt with correctly. And not repeated too often. Others are what he calls errors of "judgment." Technical errors are more often made by residents; errors of judgment are generally made by professors. Residents in surgery don't exercise much judgment. Decisions about whether or not to operate on a particular patient are usually made by the surgeons in charge of the case. Errors in those decisions can be thought of as diagnostic or prognostic, and they are usually recognized when the postoperative course is problematic. Diagnostic and prognostic errors are much tougher to pinpoint in medicine than in surgery. Probably many diagnostic errors go unrecognized. When recognized, they look bad. Patients, in accounts of their illnesses, almost universally describe trips to a series of physicians who initially misdiagnose the condition before the true disease is understood.

A third category of error Bosk calls "normative." A normative error occurs when a surgeon has failed to discharge his or her role obligations conscientiously; they are breaches of etiquette or the rules governing relations between attendings and housestaff. They are also failures by housestaff to maintain good working relationships with other health care workers and with patients' families. Normative errors make it difficult to practice good technical medicine but for seemingly extraneous reasons. Interestingly, according to Bosk, these are the errors that are judged most harshly. Technical and judgmental errors are seen as an inevitable part of life for a surgeon. A surgeon can make them and still be a good surgeon. Normative errors are seen as character flaws.

Bosk's book is about error. It discusses an elaborate mechanism by which the profession deals with errors in training and by attendings. Throughout, there is a sense that doctors are morally scrupulous, want to do what is right, are tortured by their own errors, and seek an elusive perfection. There is no discussion, in the entire book, about telling patients about errors. This is not seen as in issue.[97]

So we have a peculiar moral problem. There is a general presumption, held by most people, including most doctors, that telling the truth is a good thing. There is a further presumption, held by most people outside medicine, that doctors are not exempted from this general moral obligation. And yet, for one particular type of truth telling, involving errors in medical care, the empiric facts seem to be that doctors simply don't tell their patients the truth. Everybody seems to know it, and everybody lives with it.

The moral notion that patients ought to be told about mistakes, which seems so obvious on one level, turns out to be anything but obvious. Is that really a good idea?

Full Disclosure?

There was a terrible case in Boston recently. A thirty-nine-year-old newspaper reporter was being treated for breast cancer and doing well. During her last course of chemotherapy, she was inadvertently given four times the dose of cytoxan for four days running. She developed severe vomiting, became dehydrated, and died. The mistake was not discovered until two months later, when, partly because of the woman's journalism connections, it was written up widely in the Boston papers. How was it written up?

Bella English, a columnist in the *Globe:* "The sheer incompetence takes your breath away. It is nothing less than criminally negligent homicide. The staffers with their fingerprints on this death . . . killed Betsy just as surely as if some driver had run a stop sign and hit her" (March 29, 1995).

Globe columnist Ellen Goodman wrote: "We lost a huge portion of trust" (March 29, 1995).

There were discussions about state policies to deal with this type of error, about whether it was a "system error" or a "human error," about whether better computers in the pharmacy could have made it impossible. There were snide assertions that the Harvard doctors were more interested in research than in good patient care. The atmosphere was that of a lynching. Many of the top doctors at the hospital involved were fired. A lawsuit was filed and settled.

But who made the mistake? The order was written wrong, but other doctors were supposed to double-check it. The pharmacy was supposed to recheck it. The nurses were supposed to verify it. One safety net system after another failed, and tragedy followed. But who was really to blame? Mistakes can be recognized and interpreted only within a framework of accountability.

Mistakes happen. Disclosure isn't always benign. Forgiveness is not automatic. Doctors, reading this story, would not, I think, be more likely to disclose their next error. Disclosure assumes a certain level of trust. Lack of disclosure leads to suspicion. If doctors don't tell patients about errors, it must be because they have something to hide. But perfect disclosure is not a precondition of perfect trust.

Trial lawyers at their most idealistic think that the malpractice system is a quality-assurance system that keeps doctors honest by punishing them for mistakes. By this view, the malpractice system is a needed corrective to the pathologic secrecy of the medical profession. Bringing facts to light allows justice and improves care for all. The best doctors are rewarded and the worst are punished.

Clearly, malpractice suits change doctors' behavior. A publicized judgment in a particular case will lead doctors to do things as diverse as get informed consent, test healthy thirty-five-year-old patients for glaucoma, put newborns under phototherapy lights, and screen pregnant women for alpha-fetoprotein. Actions like these are driven by fear of punishment. Often they do not lead to improvements in care. Sometimes they lead to clinical interventions that don't improve care but only create a paper trail that will satisfy the malpractice attorneys.

In the old days, a different system prevailed. Doctors could keep their secrets and were assumed to have an interest in improving patient care. There was a psychological understanding that that interest could best be preserved if doctors were offered some sort of blanket confidentiality within which they could work with one another to correct errors and improve quality. The remnants of this philosophy exist in the idea that quality-assurance activities should not be discoverable for the purpose of lawsuits. But almost everything else is. Disclosure is now thought to be morally bracing.

But disclosure in a world where errors are thought to be compensable has its costs. Postmortem examinations have long been recognized as one of the best teaching tools in medicine. They are the final check on whether what we did and what we thought we ought to be doing were correct or whether we missed something. Today, fewer and fewer postmortem examinations are done. One of the reasons is that doctors fear they will uncover mistakes that will lead to lawsuits. The logical, self-interested response to a policy of full disclosure and swift punishment of errors is to choose willful ignorance over beneficial knowledge. We can't disclose or be punished for what we don't know.

A tension arises. Doctors are supposed to be honest. Lawsuits are supposed to help keep them that way. But lawsuits represent a system that doesn't trust doctors to be honest on their own. Such surveillance creates an incentive for doctors to be somewhat surreptitious because the system for promoting honesty is so vindictive. Rather than rewarding honesty, it punishes it. A vicious circle is set up. The less doctors are trusted, the less trustworthy they become. Instead of seeing doctors as worthy of trust, they are seen as self-serving and in need of careful policing. Instead of being guided by internal moral ideals, doctors are guided by a set of policies and regulations. Excellence is no longer internal to the profession. Instead it resides in the regulators, who are seen as morally superior. The profession becomes hollowed out.

Questions about the costs and benefits of disclosure of error must be subsumed under the larger question of the frame within which those judgments must be made. My position as a resident in the neonatal intensive care unit created a certain frame. We were involved in innovative and largely untested treatments. We were using drugs that only recently had been licensed. I was working twenty-six-hour shifts, in a position halfway between being a student and being truly accountable.

The drive for perfection is important. We strive to make no errors. The careful identification and confession of certain errors, is, in a way, an attempt to reassure ourselves that the rest of medicine is perfect. Error is seen as a small glitch in a much larger project. But what if the whole project is off course, what if we have made systematic errors that are so large and so inherent in the way we do things that we can't even see them as errors?

While I was a resident in the neonatal intensive care unit, there was a national debate about the circumstances under which doctors and parents could agree to withhold life-sustaining treatment from a neonate. The debate took place in newspapers, law courts, medical journals, and the halls of Congress. There was a sense that the customary ways of making decisions and the boundaries of parental and professional discretion needed to be reexamined. The net result of the debate was a set of agreements, some explicit and some implicit, about the goals and the methods of neonatal care. Careful restrictions were placed on the situations in which babies could be allowed to die. This was seen as a way of affirming the rights of children, the rights of citizens with disabilities, and the sanctity of life.

In many ways, the debate was a bit of political chicanery, leading pediatrics down a path that may, in the long run, be fundamentally harmful to children. We are now mandated to expend vast resources in neonatal intensive care that could, if spent in other ways, save or improve the lives of many children outside hospitals. The whole enterprise might be a big mistake that we cannot recognize or acknowledge, much less apologize for. We might be perfect soldiers in an imperfect army.

Kazuo Ishiguro's book *Remains of the Day* describes a British butler working for a man who is collaborating with the Nazis.[98] The butler seeks only to be the perfect butler, and to make the meetings with the Nazis run perfectly. His job as a butler is clear. But to the reader, the irony of the butler's willful blindness to larger events is pathetic. Ishiguro plays off the butler's political naivete and his emotional immaturity. The butler is also unable to understand or pursue his love for the housekeeper and is left, in the end, lonely and empty, an icon of a weird sort of perfection. As a butler, he made no mistakes, but his life as a man was pitifully flawed. Many doctors today seem to be in a position similar to that of the butler, working perfectly within a system that is spinning off into increasing irrelevance, sensing their own increasing irrelevance but also their powerlessness to participate in the larger events of the day. What direction should medicine go now? What are the goals? What role should doctors play? These seem to be questions that are as inconceivable as asking the butler about foreign policy.

The context in which a mistake can be recognized and judged is changing. Doctors are no longer responsible for patients in the way they used to be. Each clinical decision is scrutinized and reviewed, doctors are curtailed by utilization reviewers, clinical pathways, nursing protocols, and informed consent. Financial arrangements make them accountable to their colleagues, to large health delivery organizations, and to anonymous decision makers in invisible offices reachable only by toll-free telephone calls. The system for identifying and punishing mistakes is, in essence, a system for defining accountability, but every other aspect of current arrangements hides or diffuses accountability. One of the last remaining roles for the doctor may be as the accountable fall guy for the sins of the stockholders.

The practice of medicine necessitates a walk along a fine line between helping and hurting, between curing and killing. The enterprise is morally ambiguous to the core. Mistakes cannot be properly assessed or categorized without some vision of the larger project of which they are a part. One of the most persistent elements of human psychic life is a belief that pain and suffering are not random events in the universe but have an explanation, a meaning, a moral implication. As medicine becomes more precise and predictable, we will be better able to distinguish bad outcomes from chance. But there will always be bad outcomes.

Much of the call for truth telling today comes from a feeling that secrecy is not being used responsibly. Both doctors and patients have lost a sense of the profession as sacred and secret. There is no room for mystery. Everything is to be explicit and rational, measurable and assessable. Judgment seems to be a simple thing.

This view may work for a certain type of medicine, but for another type, doctors themselves must ultimately be accountable to define and recognize excellence and the activities that fall short of excellence. Full disclosure implies that someone else can judge, that the facts will speak for themselves. But facts are often morally mute. They can be arranged in one way or another, depending upon the context in which they are put. Judgment is the ultimate moral act, but the ultimate political act is the empowerment of judges. Doctors used to be empowered to judge their own mistakes, and this societal faith maintained a certain view of the medical profession. Today, it is unclear who should judge and by what criteria. Increases in disclosure or judgment will not restore lost faith in medicine as a profession. Instead, the illusory belief that we need full disclosure and the naive hope that we could bear it suggest the magnitude of our loss.

8

The Perils of Progress

My oldest daughter, Hannah, recently celebrated her Bat Mitzvah. As is the custom on the occasion of this coming-of-age ceremony, she read from the Torah, chanting a portion of the book of Exodus. Her passage included the Ten Commandments. After reading her Torah portion, she gave a short speech, responding to the passage she had read.

She found some of the Ten Commandments to contain easily supportable moral truths. She had trouble with others. In particular, she noted that the commandment "Honor your father and mother" presented some problems. "What should you do," she asked, "if your mother and father are just wrong?" Our extended family had gathered for the ceremony. As she spoke, I was sitting beside my mother and father. I thought of some of the disagreements we've had over the years. My daughter's question, embedded in a ceremony that affirmed ancient traditions that she was only beginning to discern and understand, poignantly embodied the perennial dilemma of youth. How do we affirm the awesome power of tradition and the wisdom of our parents, but also acknowledge the inevitable limitations of received wisdom and the need to find our own new truths? What do we do if our parents are wrong? And how do we know whether they are right or wrong?

A while back, one of the neonatologists at our hospital came to the ethics center with a problem. He was studying a new treatment for patent ductus arteriosus (PDA), a heart problem common among premature babies. His study involved the use of the drug indomethicin as a preventive treatment for premature babies who had not yet developed a PDA but who were at risk of developing one. His hypothesis was that it would be safer to treat all premature babies in order to prevent PDAs, even though some of the babies treated might never develop one, than it would be to wait until we could diagnose a PDA in some of the babies. Once diagnosed, PDAs were harder to treat, and when babies with a PDA cannot be cured with medication, they need surgery, which is more risky. Preventive treatment with the drug could avoid the need for surgery. However, the drug that he was using for preventive treatment had some known risks. It was unclear whether the benefits to the babies who would have developed PDAs would outweigh the risks to those would never have developed them in them in the first place.

To figure this out, he was doing a placebo-controlled, double-blind, randomized controlled trial. That is, half the babies got the drug and half the babies got a placebo. Neither doctors nor parents knew which babies got which, and assignment to drug or placebo group was random. Such a study is the epistemological "gold standard" for testing clinical hypotheses. It is widely believed to be the best study design for distinguishing the real effects of a treatment from chance, artifact, bias, or other misperceptions.

The neonatologist had originally planned to enroll two hundred babies in the indomethicin study. After one hundred babies had been enrolled, a preliminary analysis of the data showed that the patients treated with indomethicin seemed to be doing better than those treated with placebo. Fewer of the treated babies had died, and very few had developed the complications or side effects sometimes associated with the drug. The differences were not large enough to be statistically significant, but they were close. Instead of a p-value of 0.05, which is the widely agreed upon (but arbitrary) cutoff for statistical significance, the p-values derived from analysis of his data were between 0.05 and 0.1. This strongly suggested that indomethicin was likely to be beneficial. The question brought to the ethics committee was whether he should now continue the study, stop the study, convene a committee to review the data and decide whether to continue, modify the study, inform parents of the interim results, or what.

When our ethics committee addressed the question about the indomethicin trial, a heated discussion ensued. Some argued that until statistical significance was reached, we couldn't say that there is a difference between the two treatments or that one was better than the other. Therefore, the study should continue as designed with more patients enrolled and randomized. And there was no need to inform parents of the interim results. Because the data did not yet prove anything, we didn't know any more now than when we started the study, so there was nothing about which to inform the parents. Furthermore, parents may not be statistically sophisticated enough to understand this and may refuse to participate in the study if we informed them of the interim results. Then we could never finish the study. That would be bad because if indomethicin really is beneficial, then many other babies might suffer or die because we didn't finish a study that could convince doctors to treat them. (It would also, of course, be bad for the investigator because no journal would accept the half-finished study, and if he wouldn't be able to publish, he would have trouble getting promoted.)

By this view, the mistake had been for the investigator to look at the data. He should have had a safety committee made up of people who were not involved in the study who could have looked at the data and concluded that the study should continue. He could have been kept blissfully ignorant of the results until they reached statistical significance. This, of course, begs the question of whether continuing the study is right or wrong. Instead, it turns the moral question into a technical question, and designates a group of technical experts who have accepted the view that rigorous epistemology is a moral imperative that precedes any other.

Others in our group argued that given available information about the risks and benefits of indomethicin, and the preliminary data from this study, many doctors and parents might appropriately view prophylactic indomethicin as a preferable treatment. At the very least, it appeared that indomethicin was not contraindicated or harmful, only that it was not yet proven to be beneficial by a randomized trial. Because we allow patients to choose among many treatments that have not been proven, we should inform them of what we now know, including the results of the interim analysis, as part of a modified informed consent process for the ongoing clinical trial. If they chose to participate in the randomized study, that would be acceptable. If they chose not to participate, they would have the option to choose indomethicin or no treatment. By this view, it would be wrong to deny parents access to the information from the preliminary analysis. A doctor who did so would compromise his loyalty to his current patient so that future patients might benefit. This utilitarian view of clinical trials was thought to be morally objectionable.

As in many ethics discussions, it was easier to articulate opposing views than to come to firm conclusions. In this case, the sociology of the academic medical center predetermined the outcome. We all knew that the orthodox view was that the trial should continue and the patients should not be informed. We were just groping toward an understanding of why we felt that way or why it troubled us. In our medical culture, a certain view of epistemology coupled with a certain view of the primary importance of medical progress are foundational beliefs. We think that we know the criteria for distinguishing "facts" from mere "beliefs" and we think that there is a moral imperative to do so. The rest, as they say, is commentary.

Questions about study design and monitoring may seem like a rather arcane area of inquiry, but they cause tempers to flare. The *New England Journal of Medicine* recently carried a debate about these issues. Samuel Hellman, then dean of the Biologic Sciences Division at the University of Chicago, and D. S. Hellman argued that "randomized controlled trials [RCTs] often place physicians in the ethically intolerable position of choosing between the good of the patient and that of society. We urge that such situations be avoided and that other techniques of acquiring clinical information be adopted."[99] Eugene Passamani, a leading scientist at the National Institutes of Health, responded, "The history of medicine is richly endowed with therapies that were widely used and then shown to be ineffective or frankly toxic."[100] He cited gastric freezing for peptic ulcer disease, radiation therapy for acne, and thalidomide for sedation in pregnant women as examples of treatments that had been widely believed to be effective but either didn't work or did harm. "Physicians and their patients must be clear about the vast gulf separating promising and proved therapies," he goes on. "The only reliable way to make this distinction in the face of incomplete information about pathophysiology and treatment mechanism is to experiment, and this will increasingly involve randomized controlled trials."

The letter writers dutifully lined up on one side or the other. Ron Poland wrote, "The suggestion of [Hellman and Hellman] flies in the face of centuries of bad experience." He cited blood letting, chloramphenicol for neonatal sepsis, and the tragic experience of diethylstilbesterol (DES), a drug thought to prevent premature labor that caused cancer in the daughters of some of the women who took it. Edwin Kilbourne was astounded that the Hellmans could imply that "bias and prejudgment ought to be encouraged in a scientific study." In defense of the Hellmans' argument, Leslie Iffy wrote, "Blind emphasis on often rigid, unyielding and cumbersome RCTs is fast becoming the very straightjacket in which contemporary medical science confines itself, far too often to the detriment of original thinking." He cited Jenner, Semmelweis, and Pasteur as examples of scientists who made remarkable clinical innovations without the benefit of RCTs.[101]

The debate is more than theoretical and more than just a matter of scientific philosophy. It is about moral obligations, about money, and about the way we think of doctors and their patients. We want doctors to be scientific, but we also want them to be doctors and don't know quite how to respond when the moral values of science conflict with the moral values of medicine. The debate between the Hellmans and Passamani was about this conflict. The Hellmans were asserting the more traditional view that the values of medicine predate and preempt the values of science. Passamani was articulating a modern view, which can be interpreted in one of two ways. One interpretation is that the values of science should override those of medicine. The other is that there really is no conflict. Instead, scientific investigation is the true embodiment of the ancient values of medicine. The outcome of this debate has profound implications for the way we think about what doctors ought to be and do.

The Price of Certainty

Problems concerning randomized controlled trials come up fairly often. When azidothymidine (AZT) was first tested against placebo as a treatment for acquired immunodeficiency syndrome (AIDS), only one patient in the AZT arm of the trial died but seventeen in the placebo arm died before the study was terminated.[102] Most people, including most physicians, would have put their money on AZT after the death rate in the placebo arm reached five or ten or fifteen times the death rate in the AZT arm of the trial. Nevertheless, many scientists and statisticians thought the trial had been terminated too soon.

Baruch Brody, a philosopher and bioethicist, recently wrote a frightening book that is at least partly about the confusion between science as a methodology and science as a morality.[103] Brody tells the story of the development of thrombolytic drugs for the treatment of heart attacks. Thrombolytic drugs dissolve the clots (thrombi) that form in the arteries that supply blood to the heart. When thrombi completely occlude the coronary arteries, a heart attack ensues. In the 1970s and '80s, researchers discovered that particular drugs could dissolve the thrombi, and it seemed as if such drugs might improve survival for patients with heart attacks, especially if they were given in the first few hours after a heart attack. Because heart attacks are one of the leading causes of death in the United States and Europe, the development of these drugs was one of the hottest areas of medical research in the 1980s. It involved a number of drug companies, huge clinical trials in the United States and Europe, and ongoing controversies within the scientific community, the venture-capital markets, and the government regulatory agencies.

The story of the development and evaluation of these drugs is complex. Different companies were developing similar products. Each wanted to prove that its product was the best. Trial after trial was carried out until each company got the results needed to press its claims for the superiority of its product. Trials that showed no benefit were criticized as methodologically flawed. Trials that showed even slight (but statistically significant) benefit were publicized and touted.

As Brody tells it, the story is one of struggles for market share, of incf-ficient and intrusive government regulation, of hypocritical posturing in the financial press, and of unnecessary loss of life while patients were being denied access to proven therapy in order to serve as "controls" in studies of different drugs. "The decisions . . . to continue to run placebo-controlled trials were tragic as well as inappropriate because of the extra deaths in the placebo controlled groups" (p. 254). Although Brody clear-ly shows that the process of testing and approval for new drugs involved many considerations that were not scientific, he also documents how everything was done either in the name of science or as a cynical ruse that used the trappings of science to disguise the true motivations of the people involved. As long as it seemed to be scientific, the people involved could declare they were acting both rationally and virtuously.

The moral problems that the investigators faced in trials of throm-bolytic drugs were similar to those faced by the neonatologist at our institution. They were similar to the problem faced by Hannah at her Bat Mitzvah. How do we know for sure when to abandon the past and embrace the future, when to replace the standard and conventional approach to a problem with an innovation that seems better but that may lead to unforeseen problems? How do we ever know that a drug really works? Or if we can't know for sure, how do we decide when we are cer-tain enough?

Hannah's Bat Mitzvah was a lovely event, joyous and profoundly mov-ing. It was also expensive. So I was happy when, shortly afterward, I got a call from a drug company asking if I could give a talk at a meeting it was hosting. The meeting was about a topic I knew little about, but I needed the money and decided that I could learn. The company was developing a drug for the treatment of severe infections. The drug had looked quite promising in the lab but was not doing so well in clinical trials. As a result, many investigators were losing enthusiasm and were no longer actively enrolling patients in the clinical trial, which was beginning to stall. The company had invested a lot of money in the drug and badly wanted to finish the trial. Previous, expensive trials had shown no benefit and it was hoping that this one would salvage the FDA approval that it needed in order to recoup its investments. It decided to have a little pep rally for the investigators at a fancy resort hotel and thought a discussion of ethics would be an enjoyable and innocuous addition to the program.

The more I read about the drug and similar drugs, the more convinced I became that they were not going to be of much clinical benefit. Researchers were trying the drugs in new and different combinations, for new and different indications, but could not show improvements in patient outcome. I wondered about science and faith, about the decisions that people have to make when they pursue a line of inquiry, even though initial results are unpromising. Why do some keep going while others give up and drop out? How many dead-end roads has science gone down, and how many tortuous paths that seemed to be dead ends but eventually led to something?

On the way to the meeting, I read a *New Yorker* article by Jonathan Raban about the construction of a railroad line through Montana in 1907 and 1908.[104] One of the problems that the railroad companies faced was that they needed settlers along the route in order to service the trains and farmers to ship things by rail. But nobody wanted to live in Montana. So the companies engaged in a two-pronged strategy to induce settlers to move to Montana. One stratagem was an advertising campaign, using glossy and somewhat deceitful brochures to tout the beauty and fertility of Montana farmland. "The pamphlets were distributed by railroad agents all over the United States and Europe. They were translated into German, Swedish, Norwegian, Danish, Russian, Italian." The other stratagem was to lobby the federal government to give free land to farmers. "The terms of the Homestead Act, passed by Congress in 1909, after a great deal of lobbying by the railroad companies, were generous. The size of a government homestead on 'semi-arid land' was doubled, from a hundred and sixty acres to three hundred and twenty." A land rush of sorts followed, followed by a drought, a depression, and despair. For most people, it was impossible to make a living by farming where the average annual rainfall was about fifteen inches. "These people came over, went broke, quit their homes, and moved elsewhere," Raban writes. "Here, on these three-hundred-and-twenty-acre plots of dust, the Western forefathers were suckered."

Reading about the combination of false advertising and government subsidies for a program that seemed to be a giveaway to homesteaders but in fact was a subsidy to the railroad while on my way to a conference about an innovative medical therapy that was not going to be very effective but was probably going to be marketed, with government subsidies, to "consumers" in intensive care units around the country, I suddenly realized what I wanted to talk about. The mythology of progress, whether embodied in ideas of conquering the West or in ideas of conquering death, shapes our national destiny. It used to be the railroads opening the frontier. Today it is medicine, conquering some final molecular frontier. And just as we channeled the subsidies through surrogate programs with the Homestead Act, supporting the railroad by seeming to support the settlers, today we support the drug companies and the research enterprise by creating a pseudoentitlement to health care that seems to support patients, as long as they make decisions by which the industry can profit. Our ultimate measure of progress, our manifest destiny, is a steadily growing gross national product.

Progress has become an end in itself, which wouldn't be such a bad thing except that progress as an end in itself has no way of evaluating itself. It becomes speed rather than direction. We can measure how far and how fast we've gone but not where we are going. We can lower infant mortality, increase longevity, and delay the onset of dementia, but how will we know when we have arrived? And what will life be like when we get there? And how do we compare different approaches to these same problems? We can lower infant mortality by providing great neonatal intensive care or great prenatal care. We can decrease mortality from lung cancer by developing better chemotherapy or by reducing smoking. We can encourage changes in diet and lifestyle or we can provide an entitlement to bypass surgery. In general, there seems to be a systemic bias toward treatments that can be marketed in profitable ways and for treatments that require doctors. Until recently, there was a bias in favor of hospital-based treatments, but that era is now over. Might the future reverse the bias in favor of doctors? We tend toward a certain type of medicine, and we measure progress in ways that validate that type of medicine. We puritanically avoid small biases but seem unable to recognize or acknowledge the large ones. But the small biases may be part of the large biases, and our efforts may thus be intrinsically tainted from the start. How, after all, can we be perfectly open-minded?

Seeking a Perfect Uncertainty

Benjamin Freedman, a philosopher and bioethicist, wrote a thoughtful analysis of the conflict between moral and epistemological obligations faced by clinical trialists.[105] He contrasted the moral obligations of the individual physician, who must try to do what is right for her or his patients, with the moral obligations of the community of physicians, who must try to do what is best for all patients. Physicians often disagree about whether a drug is beneficial or not. In the example above, some were not yet convinced by the preliminary evidence and wanted to continue the AZT trial; others were convinced and wanted to stop the trial. Freedman suggests that two types of uncertainty carry moral weight. One is when an individual doctor is uncertain which of two drugs is best. Such a doctor can clearly participate in a randomized trial without violating his or her loyalty to the patient. In fact, for that doctor, a trial might be obligatory because randomization would offer the best chance of getting the patient the most beneficial treatment.

Sometimes, however, individual doctors are convinced that a certain course of treatment is best, but other doctors disagree. Freedman calls this a state of "community equipoise." Such disagreement within the professional community also creates a moral obligation to continue a trial in order to do what is best for an individual patient. Thus, according to Freedman, trials should continue until "the accumulated evidence in favor of treatment A is so strong that . . . no open-minded clinician informed of the results would still favor treatment B."

These are rigorous criteria for deciding when a trial should be stopped. They rely on open and honest communication within a well-functioning community of doctors. But they are also somewhat circular. They beg one key question: What should determine "open-mindedness"? If we statistically define the type of knowledge that *ought* to engender certainty before we begin the trial and agree that any other level or type of knowledge ought not engender certainty, then we are mathematically defining *open-mindedness* as the willingness to entertain doubts until the p-value reaches 0.05. This is not a solution to the moral problem of trying to decide when trials should stop. It is merely a restatement of it, with an arbitrary solution.

In general, distrust of historical data is one of the major justifications for conducting RCTs. It is not enough, the argument goes, to compare the effects of a new drug with last year's data about the effects of an old drug. Unrecognized aspects of disease or clinical care may have changed. Instead, we need to take today's patients and randomize them to one drug or the other and to compare outcomes of these concurrent controls.

There are two problems with this. First, to randomize patients to drug A or drug B, a physician/investigator must be genuinely uncertain which is better, or else he or she would have to recommend the preferable drug. This state of genuine uncertainty is called "equipoise." Equipoise is a very curious psychological construct. Genuine uncertainty implies a sort of ignorance, but to be genuinely uncertain whether a new drug is better than an old drug, we need to know a lot about the new drug. We are not at all ignorant. Instead, we have a well-developed sense that the new drug is neither significantly better nor significantly worse than the old one.

Interestingly, because equipoise is a *precondition* to a clinical trial, we cannot have conducted a trial in order to achieve the knowledge that got us into equipoise. But we must have gotten it somehow. Our achievement of equipoise must rely on a comparison between what we've learned about the efficacy of the new drug and historical data about the efficacy of the old drug. But here is the problem. If we can gather and evaluate those data in such a way as to allow us to be in a state of genuine uncertainty about the relative merits of the two drugs, it must be at least theoretically possible for us to gather data that would allow us to determine that one drug is superior to the other. If historical data were worthless, we could never be in a state of equipoise because we would never have any idea how the next patient might respond to either treatment. But of course we do.

The second problem is that if historical data were truly so suspect, there would be no reason to apply the results of a clinical trial to the next patient because, when it is finished, the trial itself would become historical data and we would have to be as suspicious of those data as we were of any historical data that we chose to disregard in order to justify the trial. It turns out that all data are historical, and the only way we can make any predictions about the future is to assume some continuity between the past and the future. The difference between concurrent and historic controls is one of degree, not kind. The magnitude of that degree will always vary with the particular clinical situation. Instead of assuming that historical data are suspect, we should always assess the availability and quality of those data.

The problem is that there are many ways of knowing. One, which some call the scientific and therefore morally preferable way, tries to minimize any component of knowledge that is intuitive, nonquantifiable, or has not been validated through proper studies. Another, which is much more common and perhaps more commonly wrong, relies on a variety of perceptions, intuitions, and leaps of faith that are difficult to articulate, communicate, quantify, or reproduce. The disparity between these two ways of knowing and the moral valence assigned to each lead to fundamentally different views about what sort of activity medicine is and about the standards against which its practitioners ought to measure themselves.

A combination of forces today is leading to an increased reliance on evidence-based medicine. Part of the impetus comes from the spiraling costs of medical care and the need for methods of controlling those costs that appear to be value-neutral and thus politically insulated. Complementing these economic concerns, however, is a philosophic position from within medicine that doctors *ought* to be scientific and that medicine *ought* to be rational. The irony is that the rationality of medical science is largely superficial or illusory, cloaking a series of value choices that are apparent to philosophers, sociologists, and novelists (among others) but that are ignored or simply not noticed within the insular and isolated world of medical education and health policy.

The belief in progress is central to modern American medicine. We expect scientific investigations to lead to continuous and constant improvement in our ability to understand and treat disease. We see it as part of the natural order of things that life expectancy will go up and infant mortality will go down, that five-year survival rates will improve, and that we will be healthier and healthier. We document these beliefs in government reports that are, in many ways, our equivalent of the old Soviet five-year plans. When we generally fall short, as the Soviets did, we constantly seek explanatory villains. This belief in progress may itself be irrational, however, and the whole enterprise thus embedded with tenets of faith that are profoundly unscientific, unprovable, and even untestable. What if we aren't making progress? What if new discoveries don't lead to decreases in human suffering? What if the scientific physician is not the best physician? How do we know if our parents were wrong?

Medical Progress, Clinical Research, and Risk Sharing

Progress has always been morally problematic because progress necessitates risk taking. We like progress, but we don't like taking risks. But in order to achieve progress, some doctors will need to conduct clinical investigations in which some patients will be exposed to the risks associated with new treatments. We will never be able to eliminate all those risks. New drugs or procedures, no matter how rigorously tested in the laboratory, may have unforeseen side effects when used by human patients. A unique moral question of twentieth-century medicine, which differentiates it from most medicine that came before, asks how individual physicians ought to balance their obligations to participate in this vast, ongoing enterprise of scientific progress with their obligations to do what is best for their individual patients. One of the important functions of a scientific approach to clinical research is to provide a moral framework for understanding the perils of progress.

We imagine that a careful program of scientific evaluation of new innovations is the best way to maximize benefit and minimize risk. This may be so. In seeking balance, we have developed a set of procedures and mechanisms that are superficially rational and symbolically compelling but that, on closer examination, are quite irrational and semiotically dubious. For example, we are so concerned that our drugs be safe and effective that we have created a rigid and cumbersome system of drug approval through the Food and Drug Administration. It takes years and years and millions of dollars to bring a new drug to market. The regulatory costs of the process are seen as appropriate because the process protects people from the risks of unproven treatments. However, once a drug is proven to be beneficial for any particular indication, it is approved. It can then be used by any doctor for any other indication, including things for which it was never designed or evaluated. Thus, indomethicin has been proven beneficial for the treatment of arthritis. Nevertheless, a doctor could prescribe it for PDA, for headaches, or for anything else without any regulatory controls. The neonatologist who came to us was studying indomethicin because he wanted to, not because he had to. He could have just prescribed it.

We require much more rigorous evaluation for drugs than for devices, such as artificial joints, breast implants, or intrauterine contraceptive devices, and more for devices than for new procedures, such as reduced-size liver transplants or extracorporeal membrane oxygenation. And we require almost no evaluation of the efficacy of new diagnostic tests, which can lead to medical and social consequences, can cause unnecessary worry and unnecessary further treatment, and may drive up the cost of medicine without any compensatory benefits.

In general, we are much more willing to accept the risks of not using a new drug because it has not been adequately tested, and allowing people to suffer or die who might be helped, than to accept the risks that are associated with using a new drug. The former type of risk has no liability associated with it; the latter incurs tremendous risks of tort liability.

Clearly, this system is driven as much by economics, politics, and moral symbolism as by a rational analysis of the best safeguards for patients or the moral values that we seek to embody in a regulatory system. Put another way, within a framework that appears to be rational, we have embedded structures more notable for an idiosyncratic and irrational symbolism than for a clear, concise, and consistent direction and purpose. This dual nature of medical science is apparent on the macro level in law, policy, and regulation and also on the micro level in the design of clinical trials.

One general problem with randomized trials is their embedded suspicion about the role of patients' beliefs about medicine and healing. In general, *blinded* studies are considered preferable to *unblinded* studies. This preference suggests that if the patient or the doctor knows which therapy is being given, biases may be introduced into the study. We want to isolate the pure effect of the treatment from effects that might be just in the patient's mind. This commonly held assumption betrays a peculiar view of the role of beliefs. If it is true that beliefs affect outcomes in measurable ways, then a more scientific approach would be to study the effect and try to elucidate the mechanism for it. If our beliefs have no real measurable effect on outcomes, then it shouldn't matter whether physicians or patients are aware of the treatment they are receiving. Present attitudes toward blinding suggest that we believe that a person's knowledge of treatment can affect outcome, but we don't find the effect to be worthy of scientific scrutiny. But we could study it.

Suppose we wanted to test drug A and drug B in a way that would tell both which drug was better and whether knowing which drug you were getting improved outcomes. Patients could be initially randomized into two groups. Members of one group would be allowed to choose whether they were to be given drug A or drug B, and they and their doctors would know what they were taking. Members of the other group would agree to be blinded and randomized. We could then compare the results of the two trials to see whether, in fact, blinding and randomization led to different results. If the results were better in one group than in the other, it would be interesting to see which results were better. It may be that knowing what you are taking improves outcomes. If there were not differences between the groups, it might suggest that study designs that keep people blinded and randomized may not be worth the effort.

It seems likely that the value of blinding and randomization may vary with the clinical situation. The more precisely and objectively we can measure eligibility criteria and outcomes, the less we should be concerned about bias, and the less important randomization and blinding might be. The more vague the eligibility criteria or the outcomes, the more we should worry about it. In either case, however, blinding and randomization rely on the notion that people are essentially interchangeable. We want to assign patients to groups in ways that don't account for individual differences. We test drugs on human biologic systems. This curious view of the nature of healing conflicts with our deepest beliefs about the doctor-patient relationship, in which the individuality of the doctor and the patient is thought to be of crucial importance.

Medical Science and Medical Progress

The concerns just discussed might seem quaint, abstract, or practically irrelevant. After all, one might say, the current system has led to enormous progress in medicine. It is widely assumed that such progress is based on the use of rigorous study design. Thus, Passamani and his school, in the debate with the Hellmans, implied that the moral problems of randomized trials are outweighed by the benefits in medical progress. The implication is that but for clinical trials, we would still be using leeches to treat pneumonia. However, at least some evidence suggests that such benefits may be exaggerated, that progress often occurs outside the framework of careful clinical research, and that the framework of carefully developed research may not be the best engine of progress. The relationship between medical science and medical progress is not as straightforward as it might seem. In some cases, scientists take credit for progress that they may not deserve. In fact, much medical progress takes place in the absence of clinical trials. Two examples are recent developments in neonatology and cardiology.

Throughout the 1970s, many neonatal centers reported steadily falling birthweight-specific mortality rates. In general, the exact nature of the interventions that led to these improvements in outcome were not well defined or evaluated. Different centers used different combinations of therapy, and continue to do so to this day.

Hack and colleagues studied practice variations in seven neonatal intensive care units in 1987–1988. They showed significant variations among centers relative to rates in the use of ventilators, phototherapy, indwelling lines, and treatment of symptomatic patent ductus arteriosus.

Along with striking practice variations in tertiary care centers serving similar populations, there were also differences in outcome. There was no real attempt in the study, however, to correlate particular practices with differences in outcome; in fact, there was a sense that the data were already outdated. Hack writes, "Surfactant was not in use at the time these data were collected but is currently being widely used . . . in all seven centers." Thus, she suggests that the data might be valuable not to evaluate current practices but only to compare present practices with those in the recent past.[106] Were NICUs making progress in the 1980s? Clearly they were. Study after study showed that birthweight-specific mortality was steadily falling. What therapies accounted for the progress? Nobody really knew.

Assessment of the effects of different practices in NICUs was not a priority. Instead, there was a sense that creative use of untested but intuitively appealing clinical strategies would be beneficial. The NICU culture was a progressive culture. NICU techniques will become assessable only when the baseline rate of innovation and progress has slowed.

Another example is the development of treatments for coronary artery disease. In the 1950s and 1960s, surgeons developed an innovative technique to treat angina: indirect myocardial revascularization (IMR) The technique was to implant a freely bleeding artery into the myocardium. The procedure led to clinical improvement in some cases, but many doctors remained skeptical about its efficacy or clinical usefulness.

To document the efficacy of IMR, F. M. Sones and his colleagues developed a technique he called coronary arteriography and demonstrated that the procedure did sometimes lead to apparently effective collaterals to the left anterior descending coronary artery. The new imaging technique also demonstrated something unexpected: there were often discrete areas of stenosis in the coronary arteries.[107] This stimulated Favolaro and others at the Cleveland Clinic to develop bypass grafts to circumvent areas of stenosis.[108] Initial apparent success of these procedures led to the need for answers to a number of new questions. The most urgent had to do with the effect of coronary revascularization on the natural history of coronary artery disease, angina, and congestive heart failure. Improvements in radiology that brought about the ability to answer these questions also eventuated in the development of interventions that changed the indications for surgery even before anybody knew, with certainty, what those indications should have been. Questions about the natural history of myocardial infarction eventually led to the development of other new treatments, such as thrombolytic therapy.

With each new advance, new questions were raised that hadn't even been conceptualized before. To answer the questions, new assessment techniques had to be developed and then new therapies, which in turn needed to be assessed, and on and on. Not only was the line between standard and innovative therapy blurry; the line between assessment and treatment was beginning to dissolve.

At each stage, some people argued that controlled trials should be conducted. Several large-scale trials were, in fact, carried out. Sometimes they had surprising results, sometimes they confirmed what everybody already suspected from uncontrolled observations, and sometimes they were already irrelevant because new therapies and techniques had been developed and adopted.

If the recent history of neonatology and cardiology is any guide, there are many situations in which controlled trials are not the engine of progress. Progress, wherever it comes from, seems to be somewhat mysterious and hard to standardize. It may be the case that controlled trials are most useful when progress is slow and we need to distinguish almost imperceptible differences between treatments that are quite similar. This is what we might expect if historical data allow us to assess efficacy fairly accurately, and studies can be done only on therapies that appear to be similar. It may also explain why so many randomized trials are done on things that just don't seem to matter very much, like different antibiotics for infections or steroids for septic shock.

Regulating Progress

Our current ethical frameworks for evaluation of innovative therapy focus on the micro to the exclusion of the macro, on the discrete to the exclusion of the continuous. And they focus on the new and innovative to the exclusion of old and outdated.

Each medical innovation presents a challenge to each doctor and each patient, and to society. Because medicine is a national enterprise and, in many of its features, embodies the highest moral and political ideals of society, the ways of medicine are of broad public concern. The mechanisms for encouraging or regulating progress demand not just technical evaluation but moral evaluation as well. We must ask whether today's way of allocating the perils associated with progress best embodies our ideals.

Health and disease are not dichotomous variables, and innovation or experimentation are not discrete events. Intervention and the assessment of intervention are an ongoing process. There is no point at which a therapy magically becomes standard versus experimental, any more than there is point at which it becomes obsolete. Every innovation changes the way we view every other intervention and should force us to revise our assessment of the relative risks and benefits of every existing therapy.

This realization leads to a crucial paradox. The more we learn and the more progress we make, the more uncertain we may be about what is right or wrong for any particular patient. Every disease will be increasingly seen as more complex rather than more simple. The options for therapy will increase rather than decrease. Knowledge may not converge toward a truth but may refract a single truth into a vast spectrum of truths. The smarter we get, the less clear it will be what is best for any particular patient.

Furthermore, the more knowledge we get, the harder it may be to tell where a therapy falls on the continuum from experimental to innovative to standard to outdated. Increasingly, the distinctions will blur. Instead of describing therapies as standard or experimental, we will have to learn to describe them in terms of what we know of their risks and benefits and of the degree of uncertainty associated with our knowledge. Standards of informed consent will then reflect these empiric determinations of what we know, how well we know it, and what ongoing evaluative processes are involved in refining our knowledge. All knowledge about the efficacy of treatment will need to be collected and evaluated. The controlled clinical trial will begin to seem quaint and outdated. We are beginning to see the end of one era and the dawn of another in the debates about moral imperatives and clinical trials.

The Rituals of Progress

The mechanisms for encouraging or regulating progress demand both technical and moral evaluation. Current standards embody a profound moral ambivalence toward medical progress. As patients, we all want the latest treatments. We want our doctors to be up-to-date, on the cutting edge. As a society, we heavily subsidize academic medical centers and the research that is conducted there. On the other hand, none of us want to be guinea pigs. We don't want to be experimented upon. We are afraid of the unknown. Our ambivalence is captured in the structures we have devised for oversight of the mechanisms of progress. We badly want to believe that research can be made safe. Our mechanisms for achieving this are essentially a prayer ritual, an exorcism by naming. If we call something research, gather in a circle, and perform the appropriate rituals, we hope to appease the gods who may be jealous of our progress and punish us for it.

Research is not necessarily riskier for patients than other therapeutic endeavors. This is partly because research is much more strictly supervised than standard therapy. Complications are assiduously looked for and documented, outcomes are assessed, there is oversight. In some ways, patients in research protocols are much safer than patients who are being offered "standard" therapies. Furthermore, research is conducted on therapies that are thought to be potentially better than standard therapies. Thus, although they may have some higher risk, they may also have some higher benefit. Some patients and patient advocacy groups insist upon the "right" to be enrolled in clinical trials, clearly believing that such trials are not a burden but a privilege.

Today, there is seldom such a thing as "standard" therapy. Every innovation in diagnosis or treatment alters the indications for every other diagnostic or therapeutic technique in the field. Change is not absolute but relative. Indications for treatment must be thought of in relation not only to the disease but also to every other available treatment. Furthermore, not all research involves new and untested treatments. The use of well-accepted but outdated therapies may confer risks on patients that might be avoided by the use of newer although less-well-tested treatments.

The basis of the ethical codes that govern research must be understood in terms of traditional expectations of the doctor-patient relationship. The real risk of research comes not from the new, poorly understood, or potentially hazardous treatments. Much medical therapy is new, poorly understood, and potentially hazardous. Instead, research is hazardous because the physician who conducts research is making an ineradicable moral compromise, using the patient as a means to an end. The goal is no longer solely the well-being of the patient. The physician is also, perhaps primarily, committed to creation of knowledge. Research thus transforms the doctor-patient relationship into something other than a fiduciary relationship in which the physician's sole concern is the well-being of the individual patient.

The moral intuitions that are incorporated into guidelines for research ethics are at odds with the moral intuitions of many clinical investigators, who generally perceive themselves as acting primarily to benefit their patients. They feel that evaluation of outcomes is part of their commitment to excellent patient care and that participation in clinical trials is the best way for patients to receive state-of-the-art care. Clinical trials, by this view, do not create a conflict between loyalty to the patient and development of new knowledge. Instead, clinical trials seek new knowledge in order to benefit patients, including the ones who are in the study. The research component is subsumed under the patient-care component.

The result of all this is that current standards for informed consent are counterintuitive. We currently have the strictest standards of informed consent for innovative or experimental therapies. These are also the therapies to which the strictest safety standards are applied, so that for a randomized clinical trial, for example, a panel of experts must review both proposed therapies and determine that to the best of their knowledge there is no difference between the two. Statisticians then monitor outcomes of the therapies carefully, and if one proves to be better than the other, we end the trial and provide the better therapy to all patients. It seems a bit ironic that these are the situations in which we further "protect" patients by an extraordinarily solicitous consent process. It seems it would be more sensible to use our scarce patient-protection resources in situations like standard NICU care or the use of new cardiac procedures where practice variations are enormous and nobody knows which therapies are effective or unavailing.

The division between research and therapy artificially creates a set of activities that are thought to be undertaken with the goal of creating generalizable knowledge and subjects them to excessively rigorous standards of evaluation and informed consent, and then excuses all other activities from similarly rigorous oversight. Informed consent for research is mandatorily exhaustive, but informed consent for therapy depends on the practice style of the individual physician (who will, of course, have one eye out for litigation).

Medical science and medical practice overlap but are not synonymous. Science has made many discoveries that allow doctors to be much more effective than ever before in diagnosing and treating disease. Other scientific discoveries allow diseases to be prevented and treated without the need for doctors. These include discoveries about the role of nutrition in human disease, the importance of proper treatment of sewage or well water, and the proper techniques for food preparation, as well as advances in the design of cars, airplanes, and baseball bases. These discoveries prevent disease in a way that circumvents the need for doctors. Today, a vast public health enterprise oversees food preparation, water purity, sewage treatment, injury prevention, and many other problems. Many of the people working in this enterprise are doctors, many are not, but all understand biology and epidemiology. They are all scientists, but they do not have relationships with individual patients.

In addition to public health interventions, many medical treatments are so safe and effective that they have been taken out of the hands of doctors and given directly to the public. Medications to prevent ulcers or yeast infections, and devices to prevent pregnancy all fall into this category. Other medical treatments are routinely dispensed by nurses, physician assistants, and respiratory therapists or nurse anesthetists, although they are often overseen by a doctor. To the extent that science allows discovery of safe and effective treatments, however, the need for doctors diminishes.

There were doctors long before there was medical science. Whatever these doctors were doing, they created a profession. Science is a relatively recent overlay upon a very ancient model. When I, as a modern doctor, make a clinical decision for a particular patient in a particular situation, I need to integrate knowledge about biology, pharmacology, and pathophysiology with knowledge about psychology, communication, economics, and sociology, and with beliefs about morality, loyalty, and friendship. Scientific knowledge is a part of my decision-making process but often not the greatest part.

Generally, as a practicing physician, I am not a scientist in any sense of the word. However, I recognize that much of my authority as a twentieth-century American doctor comes from a perceived link between what I do and the remarkable scientific discoveries of the biologists. I borrow their glory. I also know that science is not seen just as a methodology or a technique for answering certain types of questions or making certain types of discoveries; it is a moral force. Doctors who carry out scientific investigations are an elite. They embody a particular moral ideal of what it means to be a good doctor. To be scientific is to be modern, pure, untainted, virtuous. Science has come to symbolize a way of life and a worldview, an end itself rather than a means to an end.

But science is quintessentially a tool, a way of answering questions or testing hypotheses. It works for some questions but not for others. Today, many doctors lose sight of the limitations of science or the need for a framework within which to determine which questions ought to be posed, and what constitutes answers. We will always need to count on some received wisdom, and to honor those who bestow it upon us. Medicine's ancestry goes back much farther than science. We owe it to ourselves to remain cognizant of and respectful toward those more ancient roots.

The true peril of progress may be the way it deforms the doctor-patient relationship. We can no longer imagine a medical enterprise that is not relentlessly progressive. Our medical education system rewards researchers, not teachers or clinicians, and in this fashion creates the mechanism for passing on the ideology of progress to the next generation and the one after. In some sense, the biggest question is whether medical progress will lead to a better world. Are the resources that we commit to progress and the compromises we make to achieve it ultimately worthwhile? How much can we turn our backs on the crying demands of today's suffering, in the hopes that we will be able to relieve tomorrow's better?

These are, of course, nonscientific questions, but scientists must hold deep beliefs about the answers in order to do their work. And they must feel the contradictions. Science embodies a belief in progress, but the validity of that belief cannot be formulated as a scientific question. The endeavor requires rules and rituals, ceremonies and customs, sacred symbols. The informed-consent form is an amulet against evil, the p-value a sacred totem. We fear that if we question these sacred symbols, we shall surely perish. But that attitude is itself unscientific.

The neonatologist continued his study. Hannah continues to question her parents' wisdom in matters large and small. So should we all.

9

Do We Still Need Doctors?

Perhaps our title question is too ambiguous. If we still need doctors, what do we need them for? If not, who will replace them? Disease and death will always be with us, and we will always need to respond. The individuals who respond will need to integrate the complex and implicit values of our society on disease and death. That integrating function is complex and demanding; it can be carried out only by people who have been initiated into its mysteries and specially trained in the proper responses. We will always need such people, whether we call them doctors, shamans, priests, thanatologists, disability-rights advocates, or whatever. But what are today's mysteries, how do we judge the proper responses, and what makes the response of a "doctor" unique?

The key question is whether our societal understandings of the proper responses to disease and death, which these practitioners need to embody, have changed in such a way that we need to reevaluate our ideas about doctors. The conception of "the doctor" that has prevailed through the twentieth century has about it a certain naivete, incompleteness, and almost willful incoherence. We want the doctor to encompass and embody both ancient moral virtues and modern scientific knowledge and technique, to maintain thorough expertise in a constantly changing biophysical subspecialty, and also to be broadly educated in general medicine, the humanities, social sciences, law, and economics. We want the practice of medicine to address broad social needs but also to be exquisitely responsive to the rights, preferences, and values of the individual patient. We want cost containment, but we don't want to put a price on life. We have sought to tame or routinize disease, to make it a technical problem rather than a moral or spiritual one, and to make healing correspondingly value-neutral. Healing, we think, need no longer be based on what we "believe." It can now rest on what we "know."

We still enjoy military metaphors. We imagine that we can "declare war" on cancer, and that in spite of the risks we might face on the battlefield, our struggle is one that can define heroism. We imagine that we can and will emerge victorious, that one disease after another will fall by the wayside under the blitzkrieg of scientific investigation. Today's major campaign is the Human Genome Project, which is often viewed as the last battlefield, the one that will yield to us the power to understand, prevent, control, and eradicate every human disease or ailment. We are relentlessly progressive, certain that our efforts will make things better and better and better. And although the technical aspects of this effort are value-neutral, the crusade as a whole is highly charged with moral fervor. Better medicine is, in a sense, a state religion. We must be willing to fight and die for it.

Above all, we don't want to acknowledge that many of the things we want are mutually incompatible. We don't want to have to choose. Instead, we create a mythical ideal called "the doctor" in whose person all dissonances will be harmonized—and we are disappointed when "the doctor" can't pull off this impossible feat. Ambrose Bierce had it right when he defined the physician as "one upon whom we set our hopes when ill and our dogs when well."[109]

Perhaps in response to our own unrealistic expectations, we begin to imagine and to become concerned that our doctors might be "playing God." This is partly a fear and partly a desperate hope. The phrase is interesting. It implies a certain conception of what God is or does, and imagines that we can now begin to be and do likewise. It has a Promethean hubris and self-flattery about it that either overestimates our own powers or denigrates any meaningful conception of the powers of God. The conceit that we are playing God is, itself, and somewhat charmingly, all too human.

Our concerns about "playing God" seem to reflect one of two things. They may reflect a belief that we can now understand and control the universe, that we have the power of God. As we unravel the human genome and begin to create and patent new life forms, we may feel as if we can direct evolution. Once we stole fire from the gods; now we steal chromosomes. Alternatively, our concerns may reflect the fear that our fledgling powers to manipulate biologic systems create moral dilemmas for which we are frighteningly unprepared. We wish we could play God, but we feel that our technical ability to do so may outpace our wisdom. In either case, the concerns about playing God suggest that we are really worried about the very human role of doctors and that our anxiety is as much spiritual as it is political or economic or scientific. We need to distinguish what we do from what God does, and we worry that the distinctions are no longer clear. We are just not sure anymore whether we want doctors to be all too human or imperfectly divine.

We are unsure on a number of levels. One of the most important is medical education. To the extent that we know what doctors are, we ought to know how to prepare them. However, our process of medical education seems to be in a continuous state of identity crisis. Nicholas Christakis recently reviewed twenty-four major national reports calling for specific changes in medical-school curricula written between 1910 and 1993. He writes,

> The reports are remarkably consistent regarding the objectives of reform and the specific reforms proposed. Core objectives of reform include the following: (1) to better serve the public interest, (2) to address physician workforce needs, (3) to cope with burgeoning medical knowledge, and (4) to increase the emphasis on generalism. Proposed reforms have tended to suggest changes in manner of teaching, content of teaching, faculty development, and organizational factors. Reforms such as increasing generalist training, increasing ambulatory care exposure, providing social science courses, teaching lifelong and self-learning skills, rewarding teaching, clarifying the school mission, and centralizing curriculum control have appeared almost continuously since 1910.[110]

Both the periodic calls for such reports and the reports' remarkable consistency in calling for changes that never seem to take place suggest that the reports are up against forces stronger than they recognize or understand. Like an ineffectual Sunday sermon, they serve to highlight problems that we know and recognize but that we seem powerless to solve. As the century closes, just as when it opened, we still have trouble training generalists, increasing medical students' exposure to ambulatory care, and recognizing or rewarding good teaching. If anything, we seem to be moving further and further from these goals, in a way that seems to defy will or intention The problems don't seem amenable to identification and exhortation. They seem to grow from a deeper root.

Melvin Konner, an anthropologist and physician, has written about medical education, including reflections on his own third year at Harvard Medical School.[111] Near the end of his book, he interviews the deans of the Harvard, Johns Hopkins, Columbia, and Boston University medical schools. They all are critical of medical education, and they all propose general changes similar to those in the twenty-four reports. They call for less specialization, less emphasis on science, and more compassionate treatment of individuals with diseases, rather than simple treatment of the diseases. Konner notes, "Men who were the bosses of the bosses of my bosses at the hospital were decrying the sort of things that went on among their underlings but were bewildered as to what might be done. It was as if K [the main character in Kafka's *The Castle*] were to read in a newspaper that the head of the Castle was disturbed by the inability of individuals in the town to communicate with it and its functionaries" (pp. 369–70). The problems are so deeply embedded in the system that they have become indistinguishable from it.

The deans' powerlessness is real. Medical education has its own internal dynamic, shaped by ingrained forces and deeply held beliefs that cause even people who don't acknowledge their beliefs to act in ways that embody both the beliefs themselves and a strange powerlessness to change themselves or their world. We say we want one thing, but we act as though we wanted something very different. We say we want a certain type of doctor, but we cannot or will not build systems to educate or reward that type of doctor or the type of teacher who might train them.

Another sign of our uncertainty about the role of the doctor is the rise of the field of bioethics. This may be seen as a sign of moral vigor; however, it also seems to suggest suspicion of the ability of the medical profession itself to define, understand, and inculcate proper moral values. Prior to the twentieth century, most works about medical ethics were written by doctors (e.g., Hippocrates, Maimonides, Percival) as practical guides for other physicians. The implicit message of such guides was that doctors alone could define the morality of the profession and that this morality grew out of the essence of what it meant to be a doctor.

Modern bioethics is dominated by nonphysicians. The conflict between an internal ethic *of* the profession and an external ethic *for* the profession energizes one of the more interesting debates in the field of bioethics. Simply stated, the question is whether medicine is primarily and intrinsically a moral enterprise, with its own internal values and norms, or whether it is primarily a technical and scientific enterprise that is morally neutral until society or culture or individual patients bring values that imbue it with moral purpose.

Leon Kass, in a series of remarkable and deeply insightful essays, argues strongly that medicine is essentially a moral enterprise.[112] He elucidates the continuing relevance of the Hippocratic Oath and other ancient Greek ideas about the nature of health and disease and about the virtues and the ends of the medical profession. These ancient ideas, he believes, still define the core morality of the profession. Today's problems, in Kass's view, derive from an inattention to these values, and today's solutions can come only from a return to them.

Edmund Pellegrino also argues for a return to and a reassertion of Hippocratic ideals. Medical ethics, he writes, "is not a matter of social convenience, alterable by political social or economic exigency or by public referendum. Any ethic changeable by fortuitous social, economic, political or legal fiat ultimately ceases to be a viable ethic."[113] Like Kass, he calls for a return and rearticulation of ancient moral values as the only hope for saving the medical profession from what amounts to a hostile moral takeover.

By contrast, many bioethicists feel that medicine is a technical, rather than a moral, enterprise. In this view, doctors' expertise is as morally neutral as that of electricians or auto mechanics, and the Hippocratic oath is a narrow, sectarian, and elitist code that represents only the particular values of a particular group of physicians. Some doctors or patients might choose these values, but there is nothing universal about them. The values that inform medical practice necessarily come from outside the profession.

Veatch and Spicer, for example, argue that doctors ought not to impose their values on patients. They think it is a mistake that "some professionals persist in believing that they can determine, based on objective knowledge and their medical skill, what will benefit a patient and what will not." Such judgments, they think, require the incorporation of values, and "clinicians cannot claim expertise in value judgments."[114]

Similarly, Brennen discusses what he calls "just doctoring" and calls for a balance between a traditional medical morality, in which the physician does everything possible that might benefit his or her individual patient, and the demands of modern liberalism, which require the physician to consider and incorporate society's economic and institutional concerns.[115] "Traditional ethical notions must be modified because doctors can no longer say the 'patient comes first,' for they must also consider the hospital, the group practice, and the publicly approved reimbursement scheme. . . . A new notion of medical ethics is needed which must take into account the virtues of the institutions of the liberal state" (p. 71). Brennen remains sympathetic to the physician but, like many other philosophers, economists, and policymakers, sees that the doctor's traditional moral commitment to do everything for each patient presents society with an infinitely large and ultimately unpayable bill for services. Such economic tensions, like the moral tensions articulated by Veatch and Spicer, lead inexorably toward external controls on the content of medical practice.

There seems to be a wide gap between those, like Kass and Pellegrino, who believe that medicine should be rooted in the internal values of the profession and those, like Veatch and Brennen, who see medicine as necessarily embedded in and accountable to a particular political society. Nevertheless, there is a common thread to all of their arguments. All see the current situation in health care as an unsatisfactory compromise of moral norms. For Kass and Pellegrino, it is a compromise of the Hippocratic norms that they see as central. For Veatch and Brennen, it is a compromise of the political values that govern all aspects of our society and that should clearly govern medicine. Each of these thinkers calls for an explicit articulation of a political and moral program that would be different from today's status quo.

Sympathetic, nonideological readers find resonance in each of these arguments. We are not happy with the way things are, but we're not sure in which direction we want to go. This combination of deep dissatisfaction and intractable directionlessness shows up in numerous public-opinion polls and, as much as anything else, ultimately scuttled the Clinton health reform efforts.[116] Widespread dissatisfaction with the present system could not be translated into agreement upon any particular set of reforms. We all clearly sense that we want and need doctors and hospitals to do something other than what they now do. We just cannot agree on what.

The Seduction of Success

Part of our problem is the seductive power of medical success. When things work, we cannot resist them. And things work today better than they ever did before. This creates a certain irony with regard to today's problems, captured in Aaron Wildavsky's 1970s essay title "Doing Better and Feeling Worse." The price of success has been high. To achieve it, we have had to reconceptualize what disease is about, what healing is about, and what medicine should strive for. In the process, we have retrofitted our conception of what doctors are and what they should do, keeping the external structure intact but completely renovating the content.

Medicine's success has depended on a view that deems personal differences between individuals relatively unimportant and biological commonalities crucial. This is an observation so essential as to be trite, but it is also the source of modern medicine's essential, proud, and incontrovertibly anti-humanistic core. In this view, individual beliefs, understandings, and stories about illness are not very important. The medical gaze learns to filter out individual differences in search of their

essential underlying biological mechanisms. Medical science deliber-
ately blurs or eradicates individuality in order to reach the true,
unbiased, reproducible truths that stretch across populations. This is
perhaps what we mean by objectivity.

The secret of medicine's success is also a clue to its failure.
Throughout history, the doctor's power has always been partly interpretive, partly interventionist. Recently, the interpretive tasks have faded in
importance. Doctors no longer learn or understand or explain the meaning of illness or suffering. Instead, they learn to diagnose and to
intervene, to cure or relieve illness and suffering. When disease cannot
be cured, or when suffering can no longer be relieved, doctors are no
longer sure what to do or whether they still have a role to play. Our
responses to disease and suffering are pragmatic and mechanical. We
seek underlying mechanisms, biological causes. We want solutions that
work, not stories that mollify.

But there was always another role for doctors, or healers, or shamans.
They defined illness and gave it meaning, even when they were powerless to intervene. That symbolic, interpretive role was itself a sort of
power. Sometimes it was itself a form of healing. Hints of this ancient
role persist in some aspects of medicine. Some doctors and bioethicists
talk of "narrative ethics," about the attempt to define the meaning of illness and the morality of our responses in reference to a patient's life
story. Some illnesses are still thought of as morally tainted, as having a
meaning that is personal and important. But such views are secretive,
apologetic, or peripheral to the central semi-official beliefs of modern
medicine, which have no room for such soft speculations.

Any attempt to formulate such dichotomies risks oversimplification or
even parody. One might respond that doctors still explain illness, that
they still recognize their responsibility to care for patients and relieve
suffering even when cure is impossible, that they still see the individual
and not just the disease. Our increasing power to cure may create difficult choices for individuals, institutions, and society, but these do not
have to be either/or choices. It is not as if we can't have antibiotics and
empathy, too. However, given limited financial, emotional, and intellectual resources, we must choose which directions and efforts we will

emphasize, prioritize, and glamorize. The obvious answer is written into the architecture of our medical buildings, the reimbursement patterns of our insurance companies, and the curricula of our medical schools. We have chosen the interventionist over the interpretive, the scientific over the humanistic. We make the choices every day in thousands of small ways, and each choice is agonizing, each represents a compromise, each takes something of value away from us. But we do choose, and we have chosen, time and again, in decision after decision, over decade after decade. Our choices reveal a pattern, and that pattern is the structure of our inner desires.

Not many doctors explicitly agree that such choices are necessary. Most would assert vigorously that their loyalties to patients go beyond curing. Few define themselves as medical technicians. Their self-conception is broader. Individually, they seek, and they believe that they have found a balance. Perhaps some have. Yet most stress that scientific progress and technical competence are primary goods. If something has to give, they would rather lose a slight bit of compassion than a slight bit of competence. Most acknowledge that the energy to maintain competence is enormous. Time and energy are limited. We can't have it all. It is thus not a conscious policy to seek an imbalance but a series of tiny, difficult, subtle, and often grudging decisions to value one way of being a doctor over another. We pay more for an endoscopy than for a thorough history and physical examination, but we do still pay for a history and examination. We splurge on operating rooms or intensive care units and skimp on the outpatient clinics, yet we still have outpatient clinics. More federal grant money is available to study the molecular biology of the genome than to study the lives and choices of people with genetic problems, but there is some money to study those lives. The net result is a system that emblazons its values in the structure of its institutions while denying those values in its heart. The deans want to change the curriculum, but they cannot. Neither we nor they can resist success.

And that's fine. That's the way it should be. It would be perverse otherwise. It would be difficult to argue that it is more important to tell the stories of people with AIDS than to try to find a cure. But this changes what we think of and expect of our doctors, and it changes the way doctors think about themselves and their aspirations. It leads to a focus on measurable outcomes, on predictable interventions, on empiricism.

A series of mutually reinforcing social, political, and moral accommodations have institutionalized the doctor's role as one that embodies the values of empiricism, quantification, and objectivity. Social responses to medicine as disparate and far-reaching as malpractice litigation (which imposes a national standard of care on all doctors in definable situations and thus obliterates the space for individualistic practice styles), the doctrine of informed consent (which defines and requires a particular type of communication between doctors and their patients), and analyses of the cost-effectiveness of medical interventions (which insists that utilities can be assigned to various life states) all reinforce the view that the doctor ought to behave consistently and in precisely definable ways. But the more consistent and precisely definable things are, the more hollowed-out the doctor becomes.

All of these social responses change the way doctors must think and act and conceptualize themselves. The doctor who must seek informed consent according to a legally defined protocol in order to provide a treatment that the patient's insurance company has approved because it is the most cost-effective, and who then provides the treatment according to a practice guideline based on valid-outcomes studies is a very different creature from any doctor who has ever practiced before, since the beginning of time.

This seduction of success is strongest for medicine that works, so it has the strongest influence in situations where effective interventions are available. Decisions about which anti-hypertensive has the best cost-benefit profile, whether to have a mastectomy or a lumpectomy, or how to organize incentives within a staff-model HMO to maximize efficiency are all amenable to such influence. And we deal with such decisions quite well.

But there is a problem and a paradox. The problem is that not all decisions are so simple. Much malaise does not fit into the model. Many people suffer in ways for which there is no effective treatment. In some cases, this is because the diseases are poorly understood and the treatments largely ineffective—arthritis, lower-back pain, Huntington's or

Hurler's or Alzheimer's disease. In other cases, it is because people don't behave the way the models would have them behave. The models assume rationality, but both doctors and patients are often irrational. They have emotional needs, they lie, they live in states of phenomenal denial, they want to make a lot of money, they are deluded, they hallucinate, they hate each other.

The paradox is that no matter how much medical progress we make, the net amount of disease and suffering does not seem to decrease. The more people who are alive at any one time, the more people who will be dying. There is no closure, no endpoint, no logical conclusion to the enterprise. Instead, there is an increasing gap between our expectations of medicine as an endeavor with an understandable and achievable goal and our growing realization that medicine is an inexorably progressive enterprise without direction, a quest without a grail.

In spite of this realization, and in spite of all the changes in medicine, and doctoring, and health care delivery systems over the past century, we still cling to the belief that there is something rock-hard and immutable at the core which does not, cannot, and will not change. We believe in some essence of a medical ethic, or of a doctor-patient relationship, or of what the profession ought to do or be. But the core of medicine may not be so immutable. Enough changes in law and science, policy and economics, bioethics and religion, and the core itself may begin to crumble.

The turmoil in the health care system today is evidence that the core is crumbling. Some respond by looking forward, others by looking backward. Some try to rebuild the crumbling edifice, others want to blow it up and start over. Either response requires a re-imagining of what we want doctors to be and do. Some of the most imaginative responses today come not from medicine, bioethics, or health policy but from fiction. A number of novelists have begun to think about medicine and the physician in new ways. The doctor is becoming a new sort of protagonist in modern fiction, and hospitals or clinics are becoming a new sort of stage set. These imaginings may form the basis for a new way of understanding what we want or need from doctors. These literary responses to the current malaise are complex; they are neither systematic nor dogmatic. All draw upon psychology, religion, science, and philosophy in illustrating the precise challenges facing doctors and describing possible solutions.

Dreaming New Doctors

The Cunning Man, Robertson Davies's last novel, presents a physician, Jonathan Hullah, who develops a new way of practicing medicine.[117] "I wanted to practice medicine," Hullah says, "but I did not want to sit all day is a dismal office with a steel desk, my diplomas on the wall in cheap frames, and a dusty bunch of paper flowers for a 'homey touch,' giving something like ten minutes each to a procession of patients with the same ten diseases—the cold, coughs, the flus, etc. etc. until I became rich and dull-witted and disgusted with myself" (p. 241). The novel presents Hullah's journey of personal development.

Hullah's quest for a medical identity began when, as a small boy, he got scarlet fever in the small northern Canadian town where his parents had settled. There were two medical practitioners in town. One, Doc Ogg, was a bumbling, alcoholic, general practitioner whose primary business was selling liquor in patent medicine bottles. The other, Mrs. Smoke, was an Indian wise woman who "prepared decoctions of foxglove for weary old hearts, and doubtless sometimes hastened a death that was already on its way, or brews of deadly nightshade for palsy and epilepsy, and for a well-established cancer" (p. 37). After Ogg declared Hullah's condition terminal, Mrs. Smoke set up a tent on Hullah's lawn and disappeared into it at dusk.

"Not a sound or a sign of life came from the tent, until about ten o'clock, when bird-calls began to be heard from time to time. Bird-calls, on a night in the dead of winter, what could that be? After a time the bird-calls were intermingled with low animal cries, in which the howl of a wolf, not at full strength but low and at a great distance, was predominant. And then the tent began to shake, and it shook and it shook as if it would fly into the air. . ." (p. 27). The next morning, Hullah was cured.

Hullah liked to visit both Doc Ogg and Mrs. Smoke. Ogg told him, "Science, Jon; science rules the world. . . . I suppose innocent people have to be told what they can understand, or think they understand. They can understand miracles a lot better than they can understand science, because science takes brains. Hitch your wagon to science" (p. 45). Mrs. Smoke told him that, in order to become a healer, "you have to go crazy, starve, sweat nearly to death" (p. 41).

Hullah eventually becomes a doctor. Posted in England during World War II, he finds himself treating Canadians who have been wounded by "friendly fire" from other Canadians. "Several of these men were legless, or had lost an arm, or now had a plate in the skull. The remainder were in various stages of what used to be called 'shell-shock.' All were in bad psychological condition and many were of the group dismissed by the unthinking as 'bed-wetters.' What was I to do?" (p. 222)

These men were the casualties of both modern war and modern medicine. In both cases, they had been wounded by those who were supposed to be on their side. Their resentment knew no bounds.

Hullah began by listening to them, in talk sessions, three times a week, "accepting whatever role the rage of these men imposed on me." In a sense, he was learning to become a doctor for the incurable by listening to them tell him what they wanted him to be and then not refusing to become that thing. "I was the stupid artillery. I was the ungrateful Europe that took the best of a man's life and gave nothing in return. I was the girlfriend who did not want a crippled husband. I was the doc who couldn't solve an insoluble problem" (p. 223). In this role, Hullah was also swimming against the strong moral and pragmatic current of twentieth-century medicine, which demands that the doctor define the agenda, objectively diagnose the disease, and actively intervene in a standardized way with a treatment that will conquer the disease.

"I did not reject conventional methods of treatment," Hullah notes. "I just wanted to make sure they were the right ones. . . . It was obvious to me that the body is not a machine, varying only as the Ford varies from the Rolls Royce. Treatment must be intensely personal, and if it sometimes strays into the realm of the mind, there the physician must follow it. . . . I had discovered that a new or merely altered way of thinking was curative. It would not restore and amputated leg, or bring back an errant girlfriend, but it would give a new look at those misfortunes, and the new look was healing" (p. 247).

Hullah locates his work somewhere between the spiritual healing of Mrs. Smoke, the talking cures of psychoanalysis, the ministrations of a clergyman, and the showmanship of a quack. It is unlikely that outcomes studies could validate his interventions, or that molecular biology could explain them. It is unlikely that he could practice in a managed care setting, or that insurance would reimburse him for his efforts. But patients seek him out, and doctors refer him their most difficult and intractable patients. He makes housecalls. "I always poke into their bathrooms, pretending that I want to wash my hands; are they houses of shame, privies, and jakes bespeaking a disgust of bodily excretion? If there is a dining room, does it look like a room used only when 'company' comes, or is it the feasting hall of a happy family? How does the house smell? My nose is one of my principal diagnostic instruments. I can smell disease, very often. I can smell domestic disquiet. I can smell unhappiness" (p. 258). He listens. His physical examinations sometimes take an hour. He offers his patients whirlpool baths, massages, and complete discretion. His patients pay cash. All visits are off the record. Is he a good doctor? John Berger writes about the difficulty of assessing the value of the work of an ordinary doctor. "What is the social value of a pain eased?" he asks. "What is the value of a life saved? How does the cure of a serious illness compare in value with one of the better poems of a minor poet? How does making a correct but extremely difficult diagnosis compare with painting a great canvas? In our society we do not know how to acknowledge, to measure the contribution of an ordinary working doctor."[118] For Hullah, success is personal; it has as much to do with his own spiritual survival as it does with his patients' outcomes. Even the dichotomy, however, oversimplifies. His patients' outcomes depend upon his spiritual survival. He can heal others because he has thought deeply about healing himself.

In *The Way of the Physician*, Needleman notes that a central moral and spiritual problem for the modern physician is the scientific bureacratization of medicine. He writes, "The doctor of today is no longer an individual meeting another individual who needs him. . . . The intangibles of personal relationship, intuitive experimentation, and that special quality of inspired patience and watchfulness in treatment have been taken away from him. There are always lawyers, breathing down his neck ready to sue him for failing to follow 'acceptable' modes of treatment that are often actually inappropriate or unnecessary in a particular case."[119] Science can be exciting when it harnesses creativity to methodology and wrests new insights from the world, and even the process of taming scientific insights to the point where they are useful in medicine is risky and adventurous. But once the insights have been tamed, ennui sets in.

Walker Percy, a physician who contracted tuberculosis and became a patient, and then recovered and gave up doctoring to become a novelist, describes in his first novel, *The Moviegoer,* the temptations and the dangers of scientific investigation. His first-person narrator, Binx Bolling, comes from a family of physicians and once considered going into medical research. "One night I sat in a hotel room in Birmingham and read a book called *The Chemistry of Life.* When I finished it, it seemed as if the main goals of my search were reached or were in principle reachable. . . . The only difficulty was that though the universe had been disposed of, I myself was left over. There I lay in my hotel room with my search over yet still obliged to draw one breath and then the next."[120] His mind drifted from the research project and floated with the dust motes in the summer sun. He imagined a different sort of search, one that saw truth not in universals but in particulars.

Percy's scientific search leads to a sense of malaise. His other type of search leads to a sense of wonder. Where does this leave the physician-practitioner of scientific medicine? In a sense, both he and his patients, as individuals, are canceled out in the objective universe. Scientific medicine recognizes what is common in us all, not what is unique. It works, when it works, precisely because most of what we are is common to us all. Our individuality is dwarfed by our commonality. We share most of the same genes, we suffer from most of the same diseases, and we die, predictably, of the same, often unavoidable, causes. Basic biologic scientists, health-services researchers, policy analysts, and economists all recognize the inescapable truth that medical progress is only possible and health-service delivery systems most efficient if patients are treated as virtually interchangeable and physicians' behavior is confined within strict algorithms.

But if efficiency were all, there would be little need for doctors. Health scientists, medical technicians, or bioengineers of some other sort would be vastly preferable. Perhaps they are. The more individualistic medicine gets, the more suspicious it gets. Doctors who are outliers, patients with atypical diseases, and hospitals that do things a different way are all a little worrisome. They may be tolerated, but it is unlikely that they will be embraced. Or reimbursed.

Richard Powers, in his novel *Operation Wandering Soul*, locates his meditations on modern medicine at the edges of current practice.[121] The setting is a public children's hospital in "Angel City," a sprawling southern-California metropolis. With urban American children as patients, Powers can ironically contrast the redemptive promises of modern medicine with the grim realities of children growing up in a world facing an "epidemic of child abduction, abuse, and exploitation." In spite of the availability of neonatal intensive care, liver transplants, and extracorporeal membrane oxygenation, children at the Angel City charity hospital suffer from "things that remain obscene rumor everywhere else, obsolete, vanquished, nineteenth century ailments. Consumption. Botulism. Paint poisonings. Bizarre abdomen-filling parasites" (p. 20).

Powers's doctor-protagonist is a surgeon named Kraft who hopes that the craft of surgery, if practiced skillfully enough, will enable him to right some of the wrongs, to rectify some of the imbalances, and to survive in a world that seems as meaningless and mad as the traffic patterns on the freeways. With the tools of surgery and the magic of anesthesia, "agony need no longer always have the last word. One might do more than abide. Technique, intuition, and hands-on knowledge might, in some sustainable future, begin to grow almost equal to the body gone wrong. The infinite, anonymous petition laid at his door" (p. 26).

Sometimes surgery is enough. Broken bodies are restored, functionless limbs reconnected and enabled to walk. Sometimes it is not enough; technique fails before the infinite demand. But success or failure seem almost beside the point. Even the cures have a monotonous, alienating quality to them. The craft works only if Kraft can forget, while he works, that his patient is a person, only if he can deaden the part of himself that aspires to humanism. In one operation, he imagines the child to be inanimate or inhuman: "Opening a three-year-old's chest . . . something Gepetto-like to manipulating this puppet—paste, papier-maché, hanging strapped by its face to the anesthesia mask like a fish on a barb" (p. 23). In another operation, he realizes that he mustn't think about the *person* he is operating on, only about the *body*. "The trick is to disengage. He must read this beating shank of foal back into pure anatomic model. . . . The case must mean no more to him than any other in the cattle call of lives he has already decided. Should he feel its specific weight, even in theory, he and the girl are both dead" (p. 97).

This tension between seeing the *patient* and only seeing the *disease* has become a cliché, but it has become so in a naive and largely uncomprehending way. Doctors all opine that it is wrong to abstract the patient into the disease, to blur the uniqueness and the humanity of the person who is our patient. Almost ritualistically, we berate ourselves for doing it. Or, in a self-congratulatory mode, we imagine that other doctors, less self-aware and humanistic than ourselves, do it, but that we somehow manage to avoid it. We insert courses into the medical-school curriculum on the medical humanities, interviewing techniques, social science, behavioral science, or health policy, hoping to provide our doctors-in-training with some perspective. These efforts suggest that we see the process of alienation as avoidable, and we believe that avoiding it will be a good thing.

We don't seem ready to admit that this alienation is essential to the practice of mainstream modern medicine. Abstracting the disease from the patient is the source of medical power. It is absolutely crucial to the spiritual and psychological economy of the modern practitioner that he or she learn to do it. Alienation, disengagement, and a weird equanimity in the face of horrific disease is the essence of modern medical practice. Like Binx in his lab in *The Moviegoer*, we stand outside of the world and gaze upon it unperturbed. That is our power.

This stance works for modern medicine: it allows effective procedures, interventions, and the treatment of recognizable and precisely definable diseases. Twentieth-century medicine differs from most earlier medicine in that we have procedures and interventions that really do work. Immunizations prevent disease, antibiotics cure infections, anesthesia obliterates consciousness and pain. While earlier medicine may have worked, it did not work in the same way that modern medicine works. Certainly it was not tested and validated as modern medicine tests itself. Not everything that seems to work really works, and the techniques by which we evaluate the efficacy of diagnostic or therapeutic interventions have grown extraordinarily sophisticated. It certainly appears as if, within the limits of our current epistemology, medicine can lead to objective and predictable improvements for certain diseases or problems in a way that was never possible before. Quality in medicine is measured today like quality in industry. Our highest-quality hospitals run like factories, and they get the measurably best results. We have specialists and subspecialists with narrower and narrower areas of expertise, because that's what works.

This change has profound implications for the way we think about doctors, and illness, and treatment. It is interesting that our ideas about what a doctor should do or be are largely based on reflections made in a world when medicine didn't work the way it now works. Many attempts to deal with the role of doctors in the new world of medicine begin from the assumption that the fundamental basis of the doctor-patient relationship has not changed. But it has. The primary change is that the doctor need no longer espouse a philosophy, need no longer have a theory of health, need no longer have a particular vision or a worldview. Instead, she need only know how to handle the tools, how to transplant a heart, deliver a baby, or lower the blood pressure.

But for Powers, like many who write about medicine, measuring medicine's successes is less interesting or important than understanding how and why it fails. One question seems crucial. Are the failures temporary—states of ignorance that more research will dispel—or is failure written inevitably into the very structure of the enterprise? The progressive scientific mentality suggests the former, and Powers plays medicine against other worldviews that imagine history as progressive, culminating in some version of the end of days, heaven, nirvana. What, then, is medicine's worldview? There doesn't seem to be one. Kraft's favorite patient, a Laotian named Joy, ends up in the ICU, a double amputee, dulling her pain on her deathbed by reading *The Diary of Anne Frank:*

"Dear Kitty: I grow hopeful now; finally, everything will turn out for the good. Really, good!"

The Israeli A. B. Yehoshua, in his novel *Open Heart*, approaches questions about the moral core of medicine by contrasting British, Israeli, and Hindu ideas about life, death, and morality.[122] As he explicitly examines medical ideas about the soul that surface, between the lines, in the thoughts and conversations of the doctors in a Tel Aviv teaching hospital, he implicitly searches for the soul at the center of a seemingly soulless center of healing. The novel uses the contrast between rationalism, psychology, and mysticism to examine the difficulties we have in deciding or determining what works or what doesn't work in medicine. These themes all come together in the complex relationships between an internist, Levine, a surgeon, Hishin, a hospital administrator, Lazar, and an anesthesiologist, Nakash, all seen through the eyes of a resident, Benjy Rubin.

The novel is framed by two medical events, both of which may or may not have been mistakes. We're never quite sure. One has a good outcome, one does not. Both are presented with a circumspect ambiguity that leaves us, as readers, somewhat baffled. Did something go wrong? Should there be some moral censure of someone by someone else? Is this really how things happen in medicine? What does it mean?

The first event is a bizarre emergency blood transfusion. Lazar's twenty-four-year-old daughter, Einat, has contracted hepatitis on a trip to India. She is quite ill. Lazar wants Dr. Hishin, the chief of surgery, to accompany him on the trip to India to bring her home, but Hishin is too busy and recommends that Dr. Rubin go instead. Rubin, a mercilessly ambitious resident, can't decide whether going will be good or bad for his career. He is afraid that leaving the hospital will hurt his chances for promotion, but he also doesn't want to alienate the powerful hospital CEO. He grudgingly agrees to go.

The trip to India takes place during pilgrimage season. Lazar, his wife, Dori, and Rubin are plunged into an exotic and confusing world in which pilgrims travel to the Ganges in order to immerse themselves in its holy waters once before their death. The Israeli medical men are baffled by the Indians' complacency in the face of death, which is neither feared nor fought against. The Indians see life as a preparation for death, and death as a welcomed culmination. In this world, medicine seems particularly paradoxical, nonurgent, ritualistic.

Einat is quite weak, and on the trip home she develops recurrent nosebleeds and faints a few times. Rubin fears that she will die and decides that she needs an emergency blood transfusion. As no reliable blood banks are available, he gives Einat a direct transfusion from her mother using a procedure he learned as a military medic that was designed for emergency battlefield transfusions. The transfusion goes smoothly and seems to help. Rubin feels confident and heroic, even though Lazar appears skeptical. "I knew that everything I did here was being registered down to the last detail, and that when we got home [Lazar] would waste no time in asking Hishin and the rest of 'his' professors if it had really been necessary to perform the blood transfusion so urgently. But I was calm and sure of myself, ready not only to justify the urgent tranfusion to all the professors in the hospital but also to demand the respect due to me for my diagnosis and ingenuity in a medical emergency" (p. 116). Afterwards, Einat looks better, her nosebleeds stop, and she makes the trip home safely.

Once back in Israel, however, Levine, an expert in hepatitis, sharply criticizes Rubin's decision to perform the transfusion as "not only completely unnecessary but also irresponsible and perhaps even dangerous" (p. 201). Hishin, the professor of surgery, isn't so sure, and says to Rubin, "I'm behind your idea, especially from the psychological point of view, and as I've often told you, psychology is no less important than the knife in your hand" (p. 150). Lazar himself is convinced that the transfusion saved his daughter's life, even though it seemed strange and unnecessary at the time and even though the chief of medicine thinks it was dangerous. One of Rubin's friends also thinks it was a crazy and dangerous intervention. As readers, we can't figure it out. Was the tranfusion a mistake or a lifesaving intervention? Was Rubin heroic, crazy, or lucky? Perhaps he was crazily heroic, or heroically lucky. Did he save a life, or merely endanger one? Who really knows what works and what doesn't? Who has the authority to judge?

The second event occurs toward the end of the book. Lazar develops heart problems and requires open heart surgery. Because he is CEO of the hospital, all the prestigious physicians vie for the honor of caring for him. A specialist from Jerusalem is brought in for the surgery. The operation goes well, but Lazar develops dangerous post-operative arrhythmias. Rubin notices them and points them out to Levine, but Levine ignores them. Perhaps Levine is right to do so. When Rubin goes to the library to read about them, he reports, "No clear conclusions emerged from my reading. It appeared that there were atrial beats that could look like ventricular beats." Both Levine and Hishin ignore Rubin's concerns.

Rubin's concerns were prescient. Lazar dies as a result of the arrhythmias, a death that may or may not have been preventable. "Perhaps the immediate cause of death had been the arrhythmia," one doctor notes, "but the deterioration in Lazar's condition stemmed from an infarct caused by an occulsion in one of the bypasses" (p. 368). As with the blood transfusion, we are left confused.

Two medical events, one at the beginning involving a blood transfusion by a young resident on the road in India, and one at the end involving a misperception by a senior clinician of the electrical activity of the heart. After one, the patient recovers. After the other, the patient dies. Were they really mistakes? Is there such a thing as moral excellence or technical expertise, and is there any relationship between the two?

Through these mysterious events, Yehoshua asks what we find at the heart of medicine, what we get to when we peel away layer after layer, when we describe events as they occur to the leaders of medicine. The more piercing his gaze, the more elusive the mystery. Things happen. People trust or do not trust one another. Doctors, like others, are narcissistic, ambitious, irrational, well-meaning. They have powerful tools and amorphous goals. For the physicians in *Open Heart*, medicine seems to be strangely impersonal and amoral. The physicians judge each other, but their judgments seem strangely arbitrary. We are left thinking that the essence of medicine will never be an objective or scientific judgment but will remain a mystery, a potentially dangerous but potentially salvational blood transfusion between a mother and daughter in a strange and mystical foreign country where we take risks to save lives while, outside, the dead are burned upon pyres along the banks of the holy rivers.

Yehoshua portrays the different specialists as embodying different views of the relationship between body and soul. Hishin, the surgeon, is convinced that there is no such thing as a soul, because "he himself had spent his whole life prying into the most secret corners of the human body, and he had not yet come across any traces of a soul" (p. 380). The anesthesiologist, Nakash, in contrast, thinks of himself as "the pilot of the soul, who has to ensure that it glides painlessly through the void of sleep without being jolted or shocked, without falling. But also to make sure that it doesn't soar too high and inadvertently slip into the next world" (p. 211).

The internist, Levine, seems less concerned with such questions and more concerned with his research and with maintaining control of his department through a regime of intimidation. He periodically has episodes of severe depression, requiring mysterious leaves of absence for long inpatient hospitalizations. The other psychiatrists in the medical center are strangely peripheral, and Lazar is threatening to close down their inpatient treatment unit and build them a community mental health center instead. Levine is an expert on hepatitis, but Hishin's attitude about hepatitis is that "there isn't much to be done in these cases. Just reassure them all psychologically. Everything's psychological nowadays. . . . Hepatitis is a self-limited disease" (p. 22).

Open Heart is a novel of scientific and moral uncertainty. Like the other medical novels, it uses the life of doctors to contrast the worldview of scientific medicine with other worldviews. Each novelist plays with ideas of myth and religion, trying to find the large movements and rhythms behind the vast societal enterprise that medicine has become. In *The Cunning Man*, Hullah's best friend is an Anglican priest, and the parallel quests of the "Man of God and the Man of Science" animate the telling. In *Operation Wandering Soul*, Joy's father is a traditional Laotian healer, "certified in cures involving the recall of a person's errant soul." In *Open Heart*, Yehoshua creates a midwife with "a fervent belief in the transmigration of souls" who sends her soul to help Benjy deliver his own baby when his wife is in labor and the midwife is unexpectedly delayed.

Through these contrasts between Western medicine and other traditions, each of the novelists tries to contextualize medicine within some larger vision. By doing so, each tries to highlight the peculiarly narrow vision of modern Western biomedical science. But each also recognizes that it is precisely the narrowness of this vision, the studied unwilling-ness to ask larger questions, that defines bioscientific medicine. It is not easy to suppress the impulse to ask questions about the meaning of ill-ness or suffering or death, but such questions cannot be answered by experiment, and modern doctors learn to ignore answers that have not passed the appropriate epistemological screening tests. By this process, whole traditions and alternative ways of thinking about the world, our place in it, and the meanings of faith and truth and health are not so much opposed as they are simply invalidated.

That vision for medicine was itself once articulated in a novel. *Arrowsmith* was written in the 1920s by Sinclair Lewis, America's first Nobel laureate in literature.[123] Set in the years before and after the turn of the century, this novel captured a time in American medicine when the profession was undergoing profound change. Biologic scientists were elaborating a new, mechanistic understanding of health and disease. Diseases were to be seen not as the products of moral or social condi-tions, but as natural forces that could best be understood in the rarefied atmosphere of the laboratory. The physician of the nineteenth century, a solid, stolid, and dull captive of tradition, would be replaced by the physician-scientist, an idealist in the German tradition, a questioner of received wisdom, a skeptic about anything that was not scientifically validated.

The novel represented a new literary appreciation of the role of doc-tors in society. In writing it, Lewis collaborated with Paul de Kruif, a bench researcher from the Rockefeller Institute, and with Morris Fishbein of the American Medical Association. He sought to portray a doctor who, "starting out as a competent general practitioner, emerges as a real scientist, despising ordinary 'success.'"[124]

Prior to *Arrowsmith,* doctors had been portrayed in novels largely as buffoons. Generally inefficacious, they would appear on the scene at times of trouble and offer little assistance; often, they were objects of scorn or pity. In some cases, they would play a ceremonial role as a vil-lage intellectual or a learned man, but they were rarely the main character of the story. By the early twentieth century, this had begun to change. Doctors began to have not only enlightened ideas but also frightening new powers, and society's decisions about the use of these powers moved doctors to center stage.

Lewis realized that the physician as clinician could never embody a rigorous and romantic moral ideal, but that the physician as scientific researcher could. *Arrowsmith* catches the transition between the old type of doctor and the new, and portrays the doctor's choices as between the old, tradition-bound medical rituals on the one hand and the new, tradition-challenging empirical investigations on the other. Lewis was the first novelist to portray this choice as paradigmatic of a set of moral choices that engaged society at large. How do we tell science from pseudoscience in a world where science defines truth? How do we sort and separate the promise and the pitfalls of progress? Can an old cultural icon, the doctor, be adapted to fulfill new cultural needs?

The tension is captured in the contrast between two medical-school professors. Lloyd Davidson makes his students memorize the same lists of prescriptions that he memorized as a medical student years before. The students love him. He inculcates a tradition, and it doesn't matter whether or not the tradition worked. Medicine was about ritual, not knowledge. Max Gottlieb, an old bacteriologist, is a painstakingly careful basic scientist. He is not popular at the medical school. Colleagues pillory him as being "so devoted to Pure Science, to art for art's sake, that he would rather have people die by the right therapy than be cured by the wrong" (p. 127). Yet he is to become the hero of the novel, Arrowsmith's mentor and role model, the ideal to which twentieth-century physicians should aspire. There is something both admirable and inhuman about his approach to disease and suffering.

These two professors, the complacent traditionalist and the idealistic biologic scientist, defined the choices available to doctors. Lewis argued that medicine's future was the idealism of science. The emerging bourgeois culture of early-twentieth-century America badly needed an idealism, and science filled the bill. Capital-driven medical science offered limitless opportunities to make money by improving the human condition. We could eliminate tuberculosis and syphilis, discover vaccines that could stop the spread of plague, and insure a clean supply of milk.

But Lewis saw the tension, too. Science was humanistic in an abstract way, but in practice it sometimes demanded a heartlessness that saw individual human lives as devoid of value, interchangeable. The most stark embodiment of this tension was the randomized, controlled clinical trial. In the final episode of the book, Martin Arrowsmith, the protagonist, goes to a Caribbean island where an outbreak of plague is killing thousands. He wants to test his new vaccine, which involves administering it randomly to half the population and leaving half untreated. The scientific rationale is plain, and Martin fights to keep his clinical trial going. But his wife, who has accompanied him on the journey, succumbs to the plague, and Martin goes crazy. The demands of science become unbearable. He abandons the study, abandons his ideals, sets up a storefront clinic in a village, and starts immunizing everybody he sees. Who cares if it works?

Previous authors had compared clinical medicine to religion, but the comparison never worked. Lewis realized that the better comparison was between religion and scientific research, that the competition was not between the country doctor and the village priest but between the theologian and the basic scientist; it was not about kindliness and caring but about truth and how we know it. Enough real truth and we won't need to worry about caring anymore. We don't need compassion for a polio immunization to work. We won't need psychoanalysis once we understand how serotonin and the other neurotransmitters create our emotions.

Each stage of medical education is designed to teach people who would become physicians how to achieve precisely this sort of alienation. The lockstep trajectory of the bioscientific catechism— mathematics, physics, chemistry, biochemistry, anatomy, histology, pharmacology—is punctuated at the halfway point by an encounter with a cadaver, which serves as the only truly humanistic element of the process. This way of educating doctors represents the triumph of those for whom the universe does not consist of ultimate mysteries to be explored, but only of knotty problems to be solved. A sense of mystery is a confession of inadequacy.

This description of the process of medical education is not offered as an original insight, or even as a critique. This way of teaching medicine is the key to medicine's success. It is a mindset that was necessary for us to learn what we know. Instead, the question I am interested in is why we are surprised when the process results in physicians who think in terms of diseases rather than patients, who prefer the narrow world of the measurable to the broader world of the incomprehensible, or who seem baffled both by the inability of medicine to respond to social malaise and by the public's increasing dissatisfaction with doctors and with a medical system that delivers unprecedented results.

The Challenge of Success

We are beginning to glimpse, for the first time, how much more challenging medical success can be to the profession than medical failure ever was. Most traditional moral and professional norms of medicine were based on the implicit assumption that doctors will not have much influence on disease. When the first effective treatments came along, they were hailed as miracles. They inspired a religious feeling that created a joyous sense of social largess. We created systems to allocate those miracles as if they were manna from heaven. Everyone must have access. No one may be denied. The treatments were not goods, or commodities, or services; they were sacred entitlements, sources of salvation. Most Western democracies have traveled this path, emboldened by the slogan that we mustn't put a price on life.

Such entitlements are a good thing. Everyone ought to have access to immunizations, Pap smears, anti-hypertensive medication, and bypass surgery. Our medical schools should train practitioners to deliver these goods in a competent and cost-effective way. And when they do, they can expect to work in efficient and organized health delivery systems, and to be evaluated by how well they achieve the measurable outcomes that such medicine confidently produces. Changes in the health delivery system which incorporate these ideas were not imposed upon medicine from the outside, but were responses to changes in the way doctors think about themselves and their profession. They are driven by doctors' own beliefs about what it means to be a scientific physician.

But the schools that are training the personnel who will deploy such evidence-based, cost-effective medical treatment cannot also be expected to train the personnel who will understand and care for the patients for whom such medicine has nothing to offer. And the graduates of those schools cannot be expected to excel at those other tasks. The tensions created by our simultaneous longing for an older notion of physician-as-shaman and insistence on a notion of physician-as-scientist create a crisis of mismatched expectations. We want to hold mutually incompatible notions of what doctors ought to be, and we cannot see the contradictions.

The tensions will not go away. Neither, I think, can they be resolved in a simple and smooth way. Instead, I think the changes force us to ask whether a single profession of medicine is big enough to hold together such multiple and disparate goals. Perhaps we are witnessing the creation of a new profession, one that bears some resemblance to previously existing notions of what it means to be a doctor but that also differs in significant ways. It is a profession that is driven by science, technology, reductionist ethics, and entitlement economics. It is a profession that symbolically embodies the widely held but unspoken notions of the sacred role of biological existence in our secular and pluralist society. It is a profession that is willingly constrained by the whimsical currents of democratic politics, that is both profoundly conservative and inexorably progressive, and that is both rigorously scientific and dogmatically closed-minded. Its practitioners will specialize in the treatment of what is treatable.

At the same time that this vast, contradictory, collective enterprise flourishes, there will continue to be, as there has always been, a need for an older type of doctor. There will be people in pain who call for comfort and whose pain does not meet the criteria for any recognizable disease. There will be people who reach the end of verifiable treatment algorithms but who don't want to die according to the palliative care protocols. Such people will not want scientists or technicians. They will want someone who has the courage and the understanding and the calling to meet someone on the edge. Such companions will always be needed, regardless of what we call them.

They may not be rewarded. They may be punished. Certainly, their task will be difficult. As Mrs. Smoke told Hullah, you have to "go crazy, starve, sweat nearly to death." We can begin to see the process by which such a shakeout will take place. The teachers who teach this type of medicine will be subtly but consistently marginalized. Primary care doctors will have less time to spend with each patient, and will be expected to administer more protocol-driven treatment during that time. Specialists will be narrowly constrained within narrow administrative structures and within fixed budgets. Mistakes will be precisely defined, rigorously identified, and appropriately corrected. Health will improve. Cancers will be diagnosed earlier. The consequences of hypertension, diabetes, and glaucoma will be postponed or prevented. We will live longer and longer.

But the success will change the essence. The essence of medicine has never before incorporated notions of objectively measurable success. It was always defined in other ways. The question for the next generation is whether the challenge of success can be met without compromising something essential.

On the Margins

I work in one of the more distant hinterlands of modern medicine, in a specialty hospital for children with chronic diseases. It is not, strictly speaking, a long-term-care facility, although some of our patients stay for six months or even a year. True to the modern notion of the hospital, we are always working to get them out. We are not a place in which to take refuge, not a place to shut out the world. We are at best a way station.

But we are not like most acute care hospitals. We care for children whose diseases are, by and large, not fatal or immediately life-threatening, but not curable, either. They are diseases that people learn to live with, and that we try, through medical intervention, to make more bearable. Many of them were fatal diseases only a few years ago. And many are diseases that are the side effects of modern medical interventions—bronchopulmonary dysplasia and short-gut syndrome in the survivors of neonatal intensive care, anoxic encephalopathy in the survivors of head trauma, graft-versus-host disease in the survivors of bone marrow transplantation. Our patients are generally not so sick that they need to be in an acute care hospital, but they are not well enough to go home, either. At least not to an ordinary home.

The children who end up with these ailments don't quite fit into the smooth and efficient flow of a private practice or the precise calculations of a managed care system. They generally need more than a fifteen-minute office visit. They are often the most expensive and the most challenging patients. And they don't fit well into the thought patterns we teach in medical school—quick diagnoses, quick solutions, take this pill, have this operation. Patients these days are supposed to either get better or die. Ours do neither.

Recently, I was caring for a sixteen-year-old patient with sickle-cell disease whom I shall call Jane. It was her ninth admission in eight months. Each time, her chief complaint was severe abdominal pain. Each time, she stayed for a week or ten days. Her pain was not completely atypical for sickle-cell disease, but it was not completely typical either. Sickle-cell patients frequently have severe pain crises, but her pattern of frequent recurrences of abdominal pain, beginning in adolescence, was somewhat unusual. Still, she seemed to respond to the standard treatment—a short course of intravenous morphine given by a patient-controlled analgesia device.

Patient-controlled analgesia (PCA) is a wonderful thing. Some perceptive sufferer noticed that there are two components to pain. One is the actual pain; the other is the fear that accompanies it. The fear is more amorphous and difficult to address. It is a fear of helplessness, of loss of control, a fear that we will whimper and cry like babies, a fear that we won't be able to bear up. When opiates are given on a regular schedule, they can make the pain itself go away, but they increase the fear. Patients watch the clock as their last dose of bliss wears off and the pain begins to recur. They know they must wait, as the pain increases, and that their doctor is far away and inaccessible, their nurse rigidly bound to follow the orders that the seemingly sadistic doctor has left behind. A regular schedule is a form of torture. Like many hospital regimens, this one was designed for the comfort and convenience of the personnel, not the patients. There are many ways to tame disease. Biology offers some; rigid sociological rules offer others. Even though we cannot always cure disease, we can always maintain order.

In a patient-controlled analgesia regimen, the patient holds the button that delivers more opiates, more relief. The patient has the power.

Jane loved that sense of control. When I walked into her room, she was lying in bed with the covers up to her chin. Her hands rested on the sheet, clutching the PCA button. Her eyes were on the liquid crystal screen that displayed her dosage and rate. I asked her how she was feeling, "Well, I'm not getting enough morphine," she said. "The last time, I got 1.5 milligrams per hour continuous and one-milligram pulses. This time, they just gave me one milligram per hour with half-milligram pulses. It's not enough. My belly still hurts. Please rewrite the orders."

I asked a few more questions about her illness. She answered with similar precision until she seemed to get bored, stopped paying attention, and said her pain was getting worse.

I examined her. Her ears were OK, throat clear, heart rate 70, with a little flow murmur. Lungs clear, ribs and sternum prominent. Abdomen diffusely tender. Blood pressure OK. Her arms and legs were as spindly as tiny saplings. She weighed only 55 pounds. I took her hand,

"We'll give you a little more morphine," I said.

She sighed, closed her eyes, and turned her head to the wall.

Over the next few days, her pain gradually improved, but she didn't look much happier. She got out of her hospital gown and started wearing snappy clothes, but she still looked sad and distant. She wasn't eating much. She said that food made her belly hurt more. The nurses and the nutritionist both noted that she had some odd behaviors around mealtimes. She spent hours studying each day's menu and always ordered large amounts of food but she never ate very much. She'd play with her food, swirl it around on the plate, even save some for later. But nobody ever saw her eating it later. They also noticed that she spent a lot of time in the bathroom. She was very thin.

I tried to talk to her about her weight and her inability to eat. She said that she was hungry all the time, but couldn't eat because of the abdominal pain. As she told me about this, she started to cry, but she quickly choked back the tears and turned to watch TV.

Jane had been doing well until about a year before this admission, when she started having frequent epidsodes of abdominal pain. Her doctor thought these were just sickle-cell pain crises, but when Jane started coming in again and again, month after month, and began losing weight, she was sent to a gastroenterologist, then an endocrinologist. She had had a comprehensive diagnostic workup. All the tests had come back normal. There seemed to be nothing wrong with her gastrointestinal tract or her hormones. Then her father's employer changed HMOs, and she got a new primary care doctor.

I was concerned that she had anorexia nervosa. I recommended a psychiatric evaluation. Her parents didn't quite understand. They told me that she just had trouble eating when she was sick, that she didn't like hospital food. At home, she loved food. She did all the shopping and liked to cook meals for the whole family. I said that teenagers with eating disorders sometimes did that.

"She is very thin," I said.

After much urging, they agreed to go for an outpatient visit at an eating-disorder clinic if I could get their HMO to approve. I bravely offered to try.

Jane was feeling better. Her IV was out, and she was dressed in the latest Gap jeans and had put on a little nail polish. She was watching TV.

"How are you?"

"OK."

"I was talking to your parents."

She stared at the TV.

"I told them that I was worried about your belly pain, about the way you're losing weight, about your not eating."

"I eat at home," she said.

"You also seem sad," I said.

No response.

"I suggested that you go talk to a psychiatrist, a doctor who knows a lot about belly pain, and eating, and feeling sad. Would you like to do that?"

She shrugged.

"Do you feel sad now?"

She resolutely shook her head no. A tear rolled down her cheek.

Jane's primary care doctor was difficult to reach. When I first called, without identifying myself as a doctor, I was told that he was not in. When I called back and said I was a doctor, I got his voice mail. When I called a third time and said it was a medical emergency, his staff paged him, and after ten minutes I was finally connected. The doctor remembered the patient, but he was not aware that she was losing so much weight. I told him of my concern that she had an eating disorder, and requested a referral to a psychiatrist. He referred me to the HMO's central office, which was a long-distance call. They didn't have an 800 number.

For another hour, I was back on the line, back on hold, back to leaving voice-mail messages, back to pleading that it was a medical emergency. I finally got to an administrator who seemed to know what she was doing. She assured me that the central office had nothing to do with these matters. The primary care doctor had to decide whether a referral was necessary.

The primary care doctor seemed a little irritated with me when I called back and told him this. He didn't want to refer Jane to a psychiatrist but thought, instead, that she should see a gastroenterologist. I informed him that she already had, and that she'd seen an endocrinologist as well. I was ready to suggest that my next referral would be to a malpractice attorney when he capitulated and agreed to approve a referral to an eating-disorder clinic. Such referrals probably take a bite out of any bonus he might get for successful gatekeeping.

The family did not keep their appointment at the eating-disorder clinic. They said the HMO had not yet approved the visit. Their primary care doctor thought Jane was doing better.

I wondered if they realized how precarious things were.

"Do you know how precarious things are?"

It was August 1996. Hospital admissions were down throughout Chicago. Nobody could figure out why. People whispered "managed care" to each other in hushed tones, as if speaking of the devil, but even admissions for things that should not have been influenced by managed care, like trauma cases in the emergency room, were down. We seemed to be experiencing a mysterious outbreak of health. The hospital was losing money like crazy.

The board of directors panicked. They abruptly fired the hospital director. Like every other hospital in the Midwest, they hired consultants from southern California who preached to us that the end was nigh, but that we could repent and be saved. Repentance required us to form a zillion committees, redraw the hospital's administrative organizational chart weekly, and learn to talk about reorganizing the "patient care sector." The director of nursing resigned. We were all given new titles and assigned new job categories, and everybody began talking about "multi-tasking."

The medical staff met with one of the eager consultants. She had a big leather briefcase, and her silk scarf matched her shoes. She asked, "Do you know how precarious things are for your hospital?"

The Democratic national convention was in town to coronate a nominee whose policies on many issues are well to the right of Richard Nixon's. Richie Daley, the mayor, was determined to be a better host than his father had been. Dr. Quentin Young, who was famous for having led the doctors at Cook County out on strike in the sixties to protest conditions at the hospital, was suing the Democratic Party for the right to protest at the convention. The Democrats had decided that this time there would be designated areas for protestors, and each group would be assigned a time for their demonstration. If there were too many groups, times would be selected by lottery. Dr. Young rejected this approach. He wanted to march right up to the doors of the Convention Center and rally for a single-payer health care system.

The *Chicago Tribune* ran a story describing how unsuccessful the protestors were at getting arrested. The Chicago police, determined to erase the memory of 1968, had taken sensitivity-training courses. Bobby Rush is now a congressman. So is Sonny Bono. Their Congress held hearings to investigate FBI atrocities against Randy Weaver. FBI atrocities committed thirty years ago against the Black Panthers in our fair city have never been investigated.

Our hospital has lots of empty beds. Interestingly, our total number of admissions is up. We admit more patients, but they don't stay in the hospital as long. We are much better than we used to be at providing care for them at home. We send children home on ventilators, and we give them intravenous nutrition through catheters that feed directly into their hearts. We give them oxygen, and gastrostomy tube feedings, and nebulization treatments for asthma attacks at home. Parents draw blood to check their diabetic children's blood glucose at home and administer their insulin shots at home. Children are admitted to the hospital for surgery in the morning and they go home in the evening. Their parents administer their postoperative care. These programs have led to dramatic decreases in hospital use.

From the hospital's perspective, these programs create a vicious cycle. They were created because hospitals are so expensive. Now that we can do more and more things at home, so that stable patients are discharged, those patients who remain in the hospital are those patients who are extremely ill and physiologically unstable. And they require more care. And their care is more expensive. So there is more incentive to keep them out of the hospital. Where will it end?

From the hospital's perspective, the "best" treatments are those that make people really, really sick, so that they must stay in the hospital for a long time. Big operations, toxic chemotherapies, dramatically invasive procedures fill the bill. For most of these therapies, the patients are passive participants, too sick to help heal themselves. Once they are able to participate, they become eligible for a different sort of therapy. They need treatments that require months of work to help them achieve a slow and gradual improvement in their mood or their ability to walk or their ability to dress themselves. These treatments just don't seem like medicine. They don't show up on television. Neither do the social workers who try to painstakingly construct some patchwork of adults who resemble a family in order to help a chronically ill child pull the pieces together and grow up, who can see how the disease and the patient may interact and how hard it might be to understand the disease without also understanding the patient. Yes, I said to the consultant, things are precarious indeed.

What would Martin Arrowsmith or Jonathan Hullah or Mrs. Smoke have said to the consultants who trooped in and out of our hospitals talking about insurance products, covered lives, risk contracts, and bonus payments for physicians who manage care by spending less? Can they help us face decisions that are the inevitable result of both biologic advances and cultural changes? Twenty-first-century medicine may be as different from twentieth- as twentieth- was from nineteenth-. Science and medical technology promise changes that will be orders of magnitude more powerful than anything we've seen thus far. We can create new genes, alter and patent new species, and diagnose potentially lethal conditions in pre-implantation embryos. The old ways cannot continue, but it is unclear what the new path should be.

In some ways, the medical science that Sinclair Lewis idealized has lost its luster and become a sort of scientism. It has become so institutionalized that it is itself a new form of dogma. Once addicted to tradition, we are now addicted to change. Students are inculcated with the ideology of progress, and patients want the latest and the newest, the cutting edge. We sense that it is not only useless to memorize the preferred treatments of the last generation, but that even the preferred treatments of today are temporary stopgaps, that we will soon understand more. We have replaced faith in traditions from the past with an even stronger, almost messianic faith in the future. We believe that someday soon, everything will work the way penicillin and polio immunizations work.

Today, just as in Arrowsmith's time, the doctor's struggles are paradigmatic of a larger societal struggle. Like Lewis, today's novelists are trying to understand just what sort of hero a doctor might be. Today, the challenges come from outside the biologic sciences, from economics, health policy, health administration, clinical epidemiology, ethics, sociology, and literature. Scholars from these areas are presenting new insights and new questions about the goals and the purposes of medicine, and they are challenging the way society thinks about doctors and hospitals. Each medical choice is difficult, and the price for individuals or institutions who choose wrongly can be quite high.

Our consultants are right. Things are quite precarious, but in ways that they can't imagine. Are we better off than we were four years ago? Or forty years ago? Or four centuries ago? If so, have doctors played a role? Medicine has solved some problems and created others. The existence of an African-American teenager in Chicago with anorexia nervosa whose care suffers because her father's employer chose a new health maintenance organization may be a sign of some sort of progress, but it is so ambiguous and troubling that we can't even begin to grasp it. And the talking cures of an old-fashioned psychotherapist may be so quaint and unquantifiable that we can no longer even think about how to evaluate them, much less allocate them.

These are troubling times. Many hospitals, especially traditional community hospitals, are closing their doors forever, unable to survive in increasingly difficult fiscal times. Other hospitals, expecially those that are aggressively managed and commodified, are attracting venture capital and paying generous dividends to shareholders.[125] Doctors are uncertain about their futures. The administrative controls for medicine and the professionals who work within it are being redesigned.

And these are the best of times. Applictions to medical school were at record levels last year. More and more people want to be doctors. Television shows and movies portray doctors and nurses as romantic heroes. At scientific meetings, we are told that we are at the beginning of a new age, that the changes of the biologic revolution will be more profound than the changes of the industrial revolution. Through the industrial revolution, we remade our world; through the biologic revolution, we will be able to remake ourselves and the selves of all life on this world. But in whose image? There is a lot of talk about new solutions, but many of the solutions seem worse then the problems they set out to solve.

At the end of *Operation Wandering Soul,* Linda, the physical therapist, wonders about the enterprise in which everyone is involved at Carver General Hospital. It seems to have gone off course, taking children off the streets and, as long as they are in the hospital, providing them with no-holds-barred, high-tech care, through unending sickness and suffering, until nobody can think of anything else that might be done. But there is almost always something else. "What dying childhood needs—so obvious, she thinks, to anyone who has been paying attention—is not another swank kid-killer like Carver. . . . It needs a larger-than-life tree-fort resort, an arcaded, terraced, gardened, courtyarded children's pavillion, with ceramic and brocade, half timber and ginger-bread cupolas, a live-in architectural anthology of hospices in the oldest sense" (p. 283). She knows it won't happen, that the hospital approach is the national approach, that we want life to be longer, not better. In the end, her prayer becomes more modest. "I want a happy ending," she says. "Make someone donate their organs, at least." Have death lead to some new life through medical ritual, some passing of the spark of life, some ritual immersion in the muddy Ganges. Perhaps there can be some altruism, some hope, some sense of community, not from the healing profession and its institutions but from the grave.

The ongoing national discussion about the future of medicine seeks solutions within the enterprise—reorganizations, new corporate entities, better health services research. These may be solutions to the wrong problems. There is no "solution" to the fact that we will all suffer and will all die. There is no "solution" that avoids the need for ongoing moral choices. In the end, we are left with decisions about how and whether to respond to those whose pain seems intractable and whose suffering seems unbearable. We can devise systems to allocate resources, but we also need to think about how we will allocate the oppportunity to participate in the discussion. We can train medical technicians to transplant hearts and supplant kidneys, but we will also need to train doctors who can think about goals, purposes, and directions.

There was a time, not so long ago in our national life, when discussion of our national health care crisis focused on problems of access. Buoyant with postwar optimism, we created an army of doctors and dentists and nurses that embarked upon the medical equivalent of the Normandy invasion. We created a national research initiative that embarked on the medical equivalent of the Manhattan Project. We imagined these projects to be finite—that once we had a hospital in every town, some doctors to staff it, and some new antibiotics to deliver in it, the project would be over, the war would be won. We bravely imagined that we could afford to devote 5 percent of the gross national product to this enterprise.

Then, there was a time when we saw the problem as one of cost containment. We put curbs on the rate of growth and controls on the number of doctors, where they could come from, what specialties they could go into, and where and how they should practice. We began to sense that the enterprise was off course, and that if we could fiddle with the incentives, we could nudge it back in the direction we wanted it to go.

But it became harder and harder to nudge. Growing industries create their own political gravity. They can no longer simply be acted upon. They act. Health care is our national industry. It draws us into orbit around it. We exist to support it. Today we spend 16 percent of the gross national product on health care. We're frightened by our own creation, and we want to slow it down, to rationalize it, to restrain it.

In today's hippest discourse, the only solution is the market. Our economists assure us that a free market it the best way to get what we really want. There is no right and wrong in the market as long as it is free. Interference, regulation, restrictions, or impositions on the market create inefficiencies, which raise prices, and then we all suffer. Desire is the only moral force, and the reasons for particular desires are irrelevant. The unexamined life is thought to be the only life worth emulating.

We tack back and forth between the ideals of equality and efficiency, between democracy and capitalism, between government regulation and market forces. We try to decide among various political solutions—managed competition, a single-payer system, employer-based systems, exclusions for pre-existing conditions—each of which has passionate supporters and equally passionate detractors, but none of which seems to scratch the surface of our discontent. There is something strangely anemic about the language of the current discourse, even as the metaphors of economic and biologic science proliferate.

Market ideologists want a libertarian freedom from government regulation, a nirvana of unfettered contract-making between competent adults. Bioethical ideologists imagine a similar world, in which autonomous patients negotiate individualized and personally meaningful treatment contracts about everything from which experiments to participate in to how they want to die. In both cases, the willful turning away from larger questions to focus on the smaller questions is troubling, but it is seen as a moral challenge. We *should* resist the impulse to tamper with markets. We *should* resist the impulse to think that we might know what is best for another person, even if the person is in pain, in despair, or crying for help. We *should* distrust larger visions.

Ronald Dworkin recently analyzed the legal and moral problems of abortion and euthanasia and developed a pithy and compelling critique of current policy. In the end, however, he backed off from imposed solutions. "I have not defended any legal scheme for deciding when doctors may hasten the death of patients who understandably want to die or of unconscious patients who cannot make that choice," he writes. "My main concern has been to understand why people hold the apparently mysterious opinions they do about their own deaths, and to show what is really at stake in the heated public discussion of euthanasia."[126] The only task available to the philosopher today is to propose arguments that seem, somehow, to be representations of what people really want. The temptation to go beyond such public-opinion surveys seems to lead only to religion on the one hand or fascism on the other. Doctors, like everybody else, have become experts at market surveys.

But if we only do what people want, how do the people themselves know what they want? Is there anything we should or should not want, or are our desires an innocent force of nature, as unpredictable and unshapable as clouds in a summer sky? We cannot all be beautiful, thin, and athletic and have perfect pitch. We will not all live to be a hundred. We cannot all have perfect babies or have babies at all. We will all age, our waistlines will expand, our skin will sag, our organs will fail, we will become weak and a little dotty, our golf handicaps will rise, and we will die. We don't want those things, and we demand of medicine that each be combated. We want, therefore we must have.

What did Jane want? Just more morphine? Or something else? What did her HMO doctor want? What did either of them want of me?

Graham Greene's novel *The Power and the Glory* is set in Mexico shortly after the revolution.[127] Deciding that they no longer need religion, the new government has banned the Catholic Church and redistributed all Church property to the poor. It is a capital offense to be a priest. Most priests have given in, married, and stopped performing clerical functions. The novel focuses on one who didn't, who traveled around the small villages of northern Mexico on an ass and continued to celebrate Mass, baptize children, and perform weddings. The police are on his trail.

He is not a paragon of virtue. Quite the contrary; he is a drunkard. He has fathered at least one child. He is skeptical of the value of the services that he performs, uncertain about his belief in God. There is something unfree, unconscious, unheroic, and morally empty about his continuing to work as a priest: "He could feel no meaning any more in prayers. Why should anyone listen to his prayers?" (p. 180). Yet when he prays, the people move together into a new a sacred space. His sins and theirs momentarily fall away. He cannot begin to explain how or why what he does works in this way.

With this tale, Greene questions whether it is possible for a government to ban religion. A government can ban the buildings, the vestments, and the outward manifestations of the formal churches, yet something still remains: a more primal urge toward sanctification and prayer and transcendence that even the most miserable sinner of a priest and the simplest villagers long for and seek, even at the risk of their lives.

There may be something like this in medicine, some core of belief or morality or practice that is ineradicable and that will persist, unchanging, beneath the surface of whatever transformations take place. And there may not.

I wondered if I'd done enough for Jane. Could I have persuaded her to go to the eating-disorder clinic? Should I have reported the case to Child Protection Services? They would have laughed at me. Jane's kind and caring parents were obviously quite concerned about their daughter. They'd kept their appointments with her primary care doctor, and he had assured them that her only problem was her sickle-cell disease. They'd been to see specialists. They were neither abusive nor neglectful. What would my allegations be, exactly? Reckless endangerment by joining an HMO? Jane wasn't my primary patient. She had lots of other doctors.

And I had lots of other patients. Nobody would pay me for what I was doing for Jane. Just the opposite. If I kept bugging the HMO, it wouldn't send too many more patients my way. It was a big one, too, and our hospital was desperate to fill its beds, eager for the HMO's business. I didn't want to go the way of the rest of our hospital administration. Jane was admitted for one week every month. If she lost too much weight, we could give her intravenous hyperalimentation and charge the HMO for that. My impulses about what was needed seemed to run counter to every obvious notion of what was good for me, what was good for my hospital, and even, it seemed, what society expected of me.

And yet, there was something about the hunted look in Jane's eyes as she watched the liquid crystal readout on her morphine pump, watched as it digitally quantified our inability to relieve some deep and nameless pain. There was something weird going on that nobody wanted to see or understand or acknowledge.

But I had done my job. I was a good doctor. Nobody could blame me for Jane's suffering. Nobody would sue me if she died. Did I have some further responsibility? To whom? For what?

Notes

1. Introduction

1. M. Lipkin, Jr., "Sisyphus or Pegasus? The Physician Interviewer in the Era of Corporatization of Care," *Annals of Internal Medicine* 124 (1996): 511–13.

2. E. Ginzberg, "The Monetarization of Medical Care," *New England Journal of Medicine* 310 (1984): 1162–65.

2. Postwar Optimism

3. M. Konner, *Becoming a Doctor* (New York: Viking, 1987).

4. S. Shem, *The House of God* (New York: Bantam, 1977).

5. D. Hilfiker, *Healing the Wounds* (New York: Penguin, 1987).

6. A. Verghese, *My Own Country* (New York: Simon & Shuster, 1994).

7. Konner, *Becoming a Doctor*, p. 17.

8. S. Diem, J. D. Lantos, and J. Tulsky, "Cardiopulmonary Resuscitation on Television—Miracles and Misinformation," *New England Journal of Medicine* 334 (1996): 1578–82.

9. L. J. Blackhall, "Must We Always Use CPR?" *New England Journal of Medicine* 317 (1987): 1281–85.

10. J. D. Lantos, S. H. Miles, M. Silverstein, and C. L. Stocking, "Outcome after Cardiopulmonary Resuscitation in Babies of Very Low Birth Weight: Is CPR Futile Therapy?" *New England Journal of Medicine* 318 (1988): 91–95.

11. S. R. Kaufman, *The Healer's Tale: Transforming Medicine and Culture* (Madison: University of Wisconsin Press, 1993), pp. 239–40.

12. H. M. Somers and A. R. Somers, *Doctors, Patients and Health Insurance* (Washington, D.C.: Brookings Institution, 1961), p. 501.

13. E. J. Emanuel and A. S. Brett, "Managed Competition and the Patient-Physician Relationship," *New England Journal of Medicine* 329 (1993): 879–82.

14. S. M. Wolf, "Health Care Reform and the Future of Physician Ethics," *Hastings Center Report* 24 (March–April): 28–41.

15. C. Geertz, *Local Knowledge* (New York: Basic Books, 1983).

16. D. J. McCarty, D. L. Schiedermayer, G. S. Custer, et al., "Equity in Physician Compensation: The Marshfield Experiment," *Perspectives in Biology and Medicine* 35 (1992): 261–70.

17. R. Dubos, *The Mirage of Health* (New York: Harper & Row, 1959).

18. B. Traven, *The Bridge in the Jungle* (1938; reprint, Chicago: Ivan Dee, 1994).

19. Verghese, *My Own Country*, p. 343.

20. J. Berger, *A Fortunate Man* (New York: Vantage, 1978), p. 124.

3. Priscilla's Story

21. K. L. Jones, *Smith's Recognizable Patterns of Human Malformation* (Philadelphia: W. B. Saunders, 1988), pp. 296–97.

22. Ray S. Bowen, Jr., "Orthopaedic Problems Associated with Survival in Campomelic Dysplasia," *Clinical Orthopaedic and Related Research* 185 (1984): 77–82.

23. J. Garbarino, N. Dubrow, K. Kostelny, and C. Pardo, *Children in Danger: Coping with the Consequences of Community Violence* (San Francisco: Jossey-Bass, 1992).

24. K. Oe, *A Personal Matter* (New York: Grove Press, 1972).

25. R. Powers, *Operation Wandering Soul* (New York: William Morrow, 1993).

4. Why Should We Care about Other People's Children?

26. A. Ascherio, R. Chase, T. Cote, et al., "Effect of the Gulf War on Infant and Child Mortality in Iraq," *New England Journal of Medicine* 327 (1992): 931–36.

27. Child Abuse Amendments to the Child Abuse Prevention and Treatment and Adoption Reform Act. Public Law 98–457.

28. J. D. Lantos, "Baby Doe Five Years Later: Implications for Child Health," *New England Journal of Medicine* 317 (1987): 444–47.

29. L. M. Kopelman, T. G. Iron, and A. E. Kopelman, "Neonatologists Judge the 'Baby Doe' Regulations," *New England Journal of Medicine* 318 (1988): 677–83.

30. R. A. McCormick, "To Save or Let Die: The Dilemma of Modern Medicine," *Journal of the American Medical Association* 229 (1974): 172–76.

31. M. C. Allen, P. K. Donahue, A. E. Dusman. The limit of viability—neonatal outcomes of infants born at 22–25 weeks' gestation," *New England Journal of Medi-cine* 329 (1993): 1597–1601.

32. W. A. Silverman, "Doing More Good than Harm," *Annals of the New York Academy of Sciences* 703 (1993): 5–11.

33. M. Benjamin, J. Muyskens, and P. Saenger, "Short Children, Anxious Parents: Is Growth Hormone the Answer?" *Hastings Center Report* 14 (1984, no. 2): 5–9.

34. M. Grumbach, "Growth Hormone Therapy and the Short End of the Stick," *New England Journal of Medicine* 319 (1988): 238–40.

35. B. B. Bercu, "Growth Hormone Treatment and the Short Child: To Treat or Not to Treat?" *Journal of Pediatrics* 110 (1987): 991–95.

36. D. B. Allen and N. C. Fost, "Growth Hormone Therapy for Short Stature: Panacea or Pandora's Box?" *Journal of Pediatrics* 117 (1990): 16–21.

37. B. Stabler, P. T. Siegel, and R. R. Clopper, "Growth Delay in Children Has Psychological and Educational Co-morbidity," *Clinical Pediatrics* 30 (1991): 156–60.

38. P. D. K. Lee and R. G. Rosenfeld, "Psychosocial Correlates of Short Stature and Delayed Puberty," *Pediatric Clinics of North America* 34 (1987): 851–63.

39. E. S. McCaughey, J. Mulligan, L. D. Voss, and P. R. Betts, "Growth Delay in Children Has Psychological and Educational Co-morbidity," *Archives of Disease in Childhood* 71 (1994), pp. 201–206.

40. G. Van Vliet, D. M. Styne, S. L. Kaplan, et al., "Growth Hormone Treatment for Short Stature," *New England Journal of Medicine* 309 (1983): 1016–21.

41. R. G. Rosenfeld, R. L. Hintz, A. J. Johanson, et al., "Three Year Results of a Randomized Prospective Trial of Methionyl Human Growth Hormone and Oxandrolone in Turner Syndrome," *Journal of Pediatrics* 113 (1988): 393–400.

42. J. D. Lantos, M. Siegler, and L. M. Cuttler, "Ethical Issues in Growth Hormone Therapy," *Journal of the American Medical Association* 261 (1989): 1020–24.

43. L. Cuttler, J. B. Silvers, J. Singh, et al., "Short Stature and Growth Hormone Therapy: A National Study of Physician Recommendation Patterns," *Journal of the American Medical Association* 276 (1996): 531–37.

44. J. F. Cara and A. J. Johanson, "Growth Hormone for Short Stature Not Due to Classic Growth Hormone Deficiency," *Pediatric Clinics of North America* 37 (1990): 1229–54.

45. F. Barringer, "Pride in a Soundless World: Deaf Oppose a Hearing Aid," *New York Times,* May 16, 1993, p. 1.

46. "Cochlear Implants in Children: A Position Paper of the NAD," *NAD Broadcaster,* March 1991.

47. R. Mnookin, "Child Custody Adjudication: Judicial Functions in the Face of Indeterminacy," *Law and Contemporary Problems* 39 (1979): 226–93.

48. J. Goldstein, A. Freud, and A. Solnit, *Before the Best Interest of the Child* (New York: Free Press, 1979).

49. J. Elster, *Solomonic Judgments: Studies in the Limitations of Rationality* (Cambridge: Cambridge University Press, 1989), pp. 134–48.

50. S. Jewell, *Pricing the Priceless Child* (New York: Free Press, 1984).

51. A. Baier, *Moral Prejudices* (Cambridge: Harvard University Press, 1993), p. 28.

52. J. S. Mill, *On Liberty* (New York: Penguin, 1985), p. 197.

53. Ibid., pp. 15–16.

5. Medical Education and Medical Morality

54. J. A. Omene, J. D. Lantos, and J. C. Ihongbe, "Alpha-1-Antitrypsin Levels in the Breast Milk of Healthy Nigerian Mothers," *East African Medical Journal* 58 (1981 no. 1): 56–59.

55. J. J. Paris, R. K. Crone, and F. Reardon, "Physicians' Refusal of Requested Treatment: The Case of Baby L," *New England Journal of Medicine* 322 (1990): 1012–15.

56. D. L. Kirp, *Learning by Heart: AIDS and Schoolchildren in America's Communities* (New Brunswick: Rutgers University Press, 1989).

57. A. Camus, *The Plague* (New York: Knopf, 1948), p. 205.

58. F. L. Brancati, "The Art of Pimping," *Journal of the American Medical Association* 262 (1989): 89–90.

59. S. Shea, K. G. Nickerson, J. Tenenbaum, et al., "Compensation to a Department of Medicine and Its Faculty Members for the Teaching of Medical Students and House Staff," *New England Journal of Medicine* 334 (1996): 162–67.

60. J. Kassirer, "Tribulations and Rewards of Academic Medicine—Where Does Teaching Fit?" *New England Journal of Medicine* 334 (1996): 184–85.

61. J. Needleman, *The Way of the Physician* (New York: Arkana Press, 1985), pp. 183, 87.

6. Truths, Stories, Fictions, and Lies

62. C. Elliott, "Where Ethics Comes From and What to Do About It," *Hastings Center Report* 22 (1996, no. 4): 28–36.

63. Medical College of Wisconsin Bioethics Discussion Forum, the Internet, December 1994.

64. J. Katz, *The Silent World of Doctor and Patient* (New York: Free Press, 1984).

65. O. Sacks, *A Leg to Stand On* (New York: Harper Perennial, 1984).

66. R. F. Murphy, *The Body Silent* (New York: Norton, 1990), pp. 24–25.

67. *Salgo v. Leland Stanford University Board of Trustees*, 154 Cal. App. 2d 56 (1957).

68. *Natanson v. Kline*, 350 P2d, 1093 (1960).

69. D. J. Rothman, *Strangers at the Bedside* (New York: Basic Books, 1991), p. 55.

70. R. Powers, *Operation Wandering Soul* (New York: William Morrow, 1993), p. 37.

71. Committee on Bioethics, American Academy of Pediatrics, "Informed Consent, Parental Permission, and Assent in Pediatric Practice," *Pediatrics* 95 (1995, no. 2): 314–17.

72. P. Kramer, *Listening to Prozac* (New York: Penguin, 1993).

73. A. Alpers and B. Lo, "Physician-assisted Suicide in Oregon: A Bold Experiment," *Journal of the American Medical Association* 274 (1995): 483–87.

74. S. Toulmin, "How Medicine Saved the Life of Ethics," *Perspectives in Biology and Medicine* 25 (1982): 736–50.

75. L. R. Kass, "Practicing Ethics: Where's the Action?" *Hastings Center Report* 20 (1990, no. 1): 5–12.

76. G. A. Annas, "Will the Real Bioethics (Commission) Please Stand Up?" *Hastings Center Report* 24 (1994, no. 1): 19–21.

77. R. Pensack and D. Williams, *Raising Lazarus* (New York: Putnam, 1994).

78. P. Simon, "The Boy in the Bubble" (New York: Columbia Records, 1991).

79. M. E. Wegman, "Annual Summary of Vital Statistics," *Pediatrics* 94 (1994): 792–803.

80. J. D. Lantos, "Leah's Story," *Second Opinion* 18 (1993): 81–86.

81. W. Percy, *The Thanatos Syndrome* (New York: Ivy Books, 1987).

82. W. C. Williams, *The Doctor Stories* (New York: New Directions, 1983), p. 124.

83. D. Bonhoffer, *Ethics* (New York: Collier Books, 1986), p. 366.

7. On Mistakes and Truth Telling

84. L. Tolstoy, *The Death of Ivan Illych* (New York: Harper & Row, 1967).

85. P. Roth, *Patrimony* (New York: Touchstone, 1991).

86. J. Katz, *The Silent World of Doctor and Patient* (New York: Free Press, 1981).

87. C. L. Bosk, *Forgive and Remember: Managing Medical Failure* (Chicago: University of Chicago Press, 1979).

88. J. F. Christensen, W. Levinson, and P. M. Dunn, "The Heart of Darkness: The Impact of Perceived Mistakes on Physicians," *Journal of General Internal Medicine* 7 (1992): 424–31.

89. Roth, *Patrimony*.

90. A. Frank, *At the Will of the Body* (Boston: Houghton Mifflin, 1991).

91. O. Sacks, *A Leg to Stand On* (New York: Viking, 1978).

92. R. Pensack and D. Williams, *Raising Lazarus* (New York: Putnam, 1994).

93. D. Hilfiker, *Healing the Wounds* (New York: Penguin, 1987); "Facing Our Mistakes," *New England Journal of Medicine* 310 (1984): 118–22.

94. J. Sarfeh, D. Gregory, and E. Ingber, letters in response to Hilfiker, "Facing Our Mistakes." *New England Journal of Medicine* 310 (1984): 1675–77.

95. J. W. Ely, W. Levinson, N. C. Elder, A. G. Mainus 3d, and D. C. Vinson, "Perceived Causes of Family Physicians' Errors," *Journal of Family Practice* 40 (1995): 337–44.

96. Andrews, L. B., et al., "An Alternative Strategy for Studying Adverse Events in Medical Care," *Lancet* 349 (1997): 309–313.

97. Bosk, *Forgive and Remember*, pp. 35–70.

98. K. Ishiguro, *Remains of the Day* (Boston: Houghton Mifflin, 1991).

8. The Perils of Progress

99. S. Hellman and D. S. Hellman, "Of Mice but Not Men: Problems of the Randomized Clinical Trial," *New England Journal of Medicine* 324 (1991): 1585–89.

100. E. Passamani, "Clinical Trials—Are They Ethical?" *New England Journal of Medicine* 324 (1991): 1589–92.

101. R. Poland, E. Kilbourne, and L. Iffy, letters in *New England Journal of Medicine* 325 (1991): 13–15.

102. M. A. Fischl, D. D. Richman, M. H. Grieco, et al., "The Efficacy of Azidothymidine (AZT) in the Treatment of Patients with AIDS and AIDS-Related Complex: A Double-Blind, Placebo Controlled Trial," *New England Journal of Medicine* 317 (1987): 185–91.

103. D. Brody, *Ethical Issues in Drug Testing, Approval and Pricing* (New York: Oxford University Press, 1995).

104. J. Raban, "The Unlamented West," *New Yorker,* May 20, 1996, pp. 60–81.

105. B. Freedman, "Equipoise and the Ethics of Clinical Research," *New England Journal of Medicine* 317 (1987): 141–45.

106. M. Hack, J. D. Horbar, M. H. Malloy, et al., "Very Low Birthweight Outcomes of the National Institute of Child Health and Human Development Neonatal Network," *Pediatrics* 87 (1991): 587–97.

107. W. L. Proudfit, E. K. Shirey, and F. M. Sones, Jr., "Selective Cinecoronary Arteriography: Correlations with Clinical Findings in 1000 Patients," *Circulation* 33 (1966): 901–910.

108. R. G. Favolaro, D. B. Effler, L. K. Groves, et al., "Direct Myocardial Revascularization by Saphenous Vein Graft: Present Operative Technique Indications," *Annals of Thoracic Surgery* 10 (1970): 97–111.

9. Do We Still Need Doctors?

109. A. Bierce, *The Collected Writings of Ambrose Bierce* (New York: Citadel Press, 1946), p. 325.

110. N. A. Christakis, "The Similarity and Frequency of Proposals to Reform U. S. Medical Education: Constant Concerns." *Journal of the American Medical Association* 274 (1995): 706–711.

111. M. Konner, *Becoming a Doctor* (New York: Viking, 1987), pp. 369–70.

112. L. Kass, *Toward a More Natural Science* (New York: Free Press, 1985).

113. E. Pellegrino, "Ethics," *Journal of the American Medical Association* 275 (1996): 1807–1809.

114. R. M. Veatch and C. M. Spicer, "Medically Futile Care: The Role of the Physician in Setting Limits," *American Journal of Law and Medicine* 18 (1992): 15–36.

115. T. Brennen, *Just Doctoring* (Cambridge: Harvard University Press, 1992).

116. R. J. Blendon, M. Brodie and J. Benson, "What Happened to Americans' Support for the Clinton Plan?" *Health Affairs* 14 (1995): 7–23.

117. Robertson Davies, *The Cunning Man* (New York: Viking, 1995).

118. J. Berger, *A Fortunate Man* (New York: Vantage, 1978), p. 124.

119. Needleman, *The Way of the Physician*, p. 87.

120. W. Percy, *The Moviegoer* (New York: Ballantine Books, 1961), p. 60.

121. R. Powers, *Operation Wandering Soul* (New York: William Morrow, 1994).

122. A. B. Yehoshua, *Open Heart* (New York: Doubleday, 1996).

123. Sinclair Lewis, *Arrowsmith* (New York: Harcourt Brace, 1925).

124. L. Richardson, "*Arrowsmith*: Genesis, Development, Versions," in R. J. Griffin, ed., *Twentieth Century Interpretations of* Arrowsmith (Englewood Cliffs, N.J.: Prentice-Hall, 1968), p. 24.

125. R. Kuttner, "Columbia/HCA and the Resurgence of the For-profit Hospital Business," *New England Journal of Medicine* 335 (1996): 362–67.

126. R. Dworkin, *Life's Dominion* (New York: Vintage, 1993), p. 216.

127. Graham Greene, *The Power and the Glory* (New York: Time, Inc., 1940).

Index

A Personal Matter (Oe), 40–41
Abortion, 195
AIDS, 72, 91, 115
   AZT and, 138, 142
   truth-telling dilemma, 83–84, 104–106
Allegheny County Medical Society, 67
Allen, D. B., 201n.36
Allen, M. C., 201n.31
Alpers, A., 203n.73
Ambulatory Pediatrics Association, 92
American Academy of Pediatrics, 90, 203n.71
American Medical Association, 26, 179
American Pediatric Society, 92
American Sign Language, 58
Anesthesia, 5
Angina, 149
Annals of Internal Medicine, 19
Annas, George, 98, 203n.76
Anorexia nervosa, HMO's treatment of, 187–188, 195–197
Aristotle, 112
Arrowsmith (Lewis), 179–180
Arthritis, 146, 166
Ascherio, A., 200n.26
Asthma, 34
Azidothymidine (AZT), 138, 142

Baby L case, medical futility and, 71–72
Baier, Annette, 61–62, 202n.51

Barringer, F., 202n.45
Barzun, Jacques, 83
Benjamin, M., 201n.33
Benson, J., 205n.116
Bercu, B. B., 201n.35
Berger, John, 30, 170, 200n.20, 206n.118
Best interest standard, 52–54
   political economy of, 60–64
Botto, P. R., 201n.39
Bierce, Ambrose, 158, 203n.61, 205n.109
Bioethics, 61, 64, 67–69; *see also* Medical ethics
   American bioethics, 42, 83
   Baby L case, 71–72
   CPR and, 15–16, 53
   current movement in, 98, 161
   death and dying, 46–47, 68–69, 119
   diversity issues and, 103
   drug/treatment clinical trials and, 134–137, 139, 142, 152
   growing interest in, 97–98
   Hippocratic norms versus political values, 161–163
   informed consent, 86–89, 90–92, 107–111
   medical futility, 70–71
   medicine as technical knowledge, 161–162

moral theory/morality of medicine, 42,
  62–65, 79, 81, 96, 101, 132, 175
narrative ethics, 164
religious beliefs and, 108–111
research guidelines, 88–89, 153
science as methodology/morality, 92–97,
  138, 178
truth telling and, 86, 122
Blackhall, L. J., 199n.9
Blendon, R. J., 205n.116
Blinded/unblinded studies, 147
Bloodletting, 43, 87
Bonhoffer, Dietrich, 114–115, 204n.83
Bono, Sonny, 190
Bosk, Charles, 123, 126–127, 204n.87,
  204n.97
Boston University, 160
Bowen, Ray S., Jr., 200n.22
Brain death, 68–69
religious beliefs and, 69
Brancati, F. L., 202n.58
Breast cancer, 87, 121, 128
  personal experience of mother-in-law,
    Evelyn, 9–10
Brennen, T., 162–163, 205n.115
Brett, Alan, 23, 200n.13
The Bridge in the Jungle (Traven), 29
Brody, Baruch, 138–139, 205n.103
Brudic, M., 205n.116
Bush, George, 49

Cadavers, 68, 74–75
  non-heart-beating cadavers, 68
Campomelic dysplasia, 32–33
Camus, Albert, 19, 76–77, 202n.57
Cancer patients, 15, 38, 44, 88, 101, 158
  breast cancer, 9–10, 87, 121, 128
  legalized euthanasia and, 45–47
  uterine cancer, 107
Capitated payment systems, 7
Cara, J. F., 202n.44
Cardiac arrest, 13
Cardiac arrhythmia, 11
Cardiopulmonary resuscitation (CPR),
  11–14, 29, 31, 34, 36
  as ethical issue, 15–16, 53
  as imagery of modern medicine, 11–14

personal tragedy of sister-in-law, 11–14
slow code CPR, 43
survival rates and, 15
The Castle (Kafka), 160
Cauna, Nicholas, 74
Centers for Disease Control (CDC), 72
Cerebral palsy, 34
Chase, R., 200n.26
Chicago Tribune, 189
Children
  abuse and treatment of, 51–53
  best-interest standard, 52–54
    cochlear implants, 57–58
    custody decisions, 58–60
    growth hormone for short children,
      54–57
    political economy of, 60–64
  Child Abuse and Treatment Act, 53,
    200n.27
  childhood diseases, 49
  chronic disease and, 34, 37–39, 44–45,
    172–173, 184–185
  current situation, 45, 64
  informed-consent and, 90–92
  life-and-death medical decisions and,
    39–42, 52
  medical ethics of treatment, 42
  rights and laws, 38–40, 50
  truth telling and, 83–85, 104–105
  ventilator-dependent patients, 32–35, 49,
    53, 71, 95
Children's Crusade, 44
Children's Hospital (Kuwait City), 49
Christakis, Nicholas, 159, 205n.110
Christensen, J. F., 123, 204n.88
Cleft palate, 33
Cleveland Clinic, 149
Clinical drug testing
  bioethics and, 134–139, 142, 152
  blinded/unblinded studies, 147
  historical data and, 144, 150
  placebo-controlled, double-blind testing,
    134–135
  randomized controlled trials (RCTs),
    136–138, 146–148
  risks of, 145–146
Clinical medicine, 181

Clinical nurse specialists, 7, 155
Clinical research, guidelines for, 88–89, 153
Clinton, Hillary, 17–18, 105
Clinton, William J., 16 18, 26, 31, 105, 163
Clopper, R. R., 201n.37
Cochlear implants, 57 58
Columbia University Medical Center, 77, 160
Community equipoise, 142–143
Confidentiality, 8
Congenital anomalies, 52
Coronary artery disease, 149
Corporatization of health care, 3
Cote, T., 200n.26
Crone, R. K., 202n.55
The Cunning Man (Davies), 168–170, 178
Custer, G. S., 200n.16
Custody decisions, child's best interest and, 58–60
Cuttler, L. M., 201n.42, 201n.43

Daley, Richard, 189
Davies, Robertson, 168, 206n.117
De Kruif, Paul, 179
Death; *see also* Euthanasia
  bioethics and, 119
  brain death, 68–69
  childhood death, 39
  do-not-resuscitate orders, 33–36, 43, 112
  infant mortality rates, 49, 67, 103, 141, 148 149
  lethal injection, 95
  modern medicine and, 29 31
  non-heart-beating cadavers, 68
  physician-assisted death, 43, 46–47, 94–95
  tragedy of Bethann (sister-in-law), 10–12, 28–30
The Death of Ivan Illych (Tolstoy), 120
Democratic National Convention, 189–190
Detre, Thomas, 73
Diabetes, 34
Diarrhea, 30, 67, 75
Diem, S., 199n.8
Diphtheria, 49, 67
Diversity issues, 103, 141–142
Do-not-resuscitate orders, 33–36, 43, 112

Doctor-patient relationship, 2, 4, 6–7, 22–23; *see also* Children
  best treatment dilemma, 88, 107–110
  best interest standard and, 60–61
  children/young patients and, 11, 39, 90–92, 104
  clinical trials and, 148, 153
  communication and, 122–123
  disease, as personal tragedy, 9–10, 173–174
  doctor as patient, 99–100
  group practices and, 22
  informed consent, 86–87, 89
  medical progress and, 152–156
  truth telling, 82–84, 104–106, 114–115, 120
    historical context, 86–90
    tradition of withholding truth, 85
Doctors
  clinical drug/treatment trials and, 142
  do-no-harm standard, 87
  errors and mistakes, 118–119, 121, 123–124, 126–128
    accountability, 131–132
    disclosure of, 128–132
  fictionalized portrayals, 15, 168–182
    Arrowsmith (Lewis) and modern medicine, 179–181, 191
    The Cunning Man (Davies) as a new practitioner, 168–170
    The Moviegoer (Percy) and scientific research, 171, 173
    Open Heart (Yehoshua) and the moral core of medicine, 175–178
    Operation Wandering Soul (Powers) and meditations on modern medicine, 172–174
    The Way of the Physician (Needleman) and scientific bureaucracy, 170–171
  as God, 159
  as healer, 4–5, 78, 164
  moral dilemmas of, 79, 113–115
  need for, 1–2, 157–158
  role of, 1, 4, 6–7, 30, 76, 131–132, 165–166
  as scientist, 4–5, 9, 27, 137, 155–156,

171, 183
specialization and, 7, 9, 21–22, 25
technical knowledge and, 161–162
value of work, 30–31, 113–114
"Doing Better and Feeling Worse"
(Wildavsky), 163
Donahue, P. K., 201n.31
Downs syndrome, 116
Drug testing and clinical trials, 134–139,
142, 152; *see also* Clinical drug test-
ing
Dubos, René, 28, 200n.17
Dubrow, N., 200n.23
Dunn, P. M., 204n.88
Dusman, A. E., 201n.31
Dwarfing syndrome, 32
Dworkin, Ronald, 195, 206n.126

East African Medical Journal, 67
Effler, D. B., 205n.108
Elder, N. C., 204n.95
Electrocardiograms, 23
Elliot, Carl, 82, 203n.62
Elster, Jon, 59, 202n.49
Ely, J. W., 125, 204n.95
Emanuel, Ezekiel, 23, 200n.13
Emphysema, personal experience of father-
in-law, 9–10
English, Bella, 128
Equipoise, 142–143
Errors and mistakes, 116–119
accountability and, 131–132
definition of, 125–127
diagnostic and prognostic errors, 127
disclosure of, 128–132
eyebrow-raising events, 126
judgment error, 127
moral evasion, 119–122
normative error, 127
system error, 128
technical error, 127
E.T., 14
Ethics (Bonhoffer), 114–115
Euthanasia, 68, 95, 97, 112, 195
legalization of, 45–47
Eyebrow-raising events, 126
"Facing Our Mistakes" (Hilfiker), 124

Family practice, 19
Favolaro, R. G., 149, 205n.108
Fischl, M. A., 205n.102
Fishbein, Morris, 179
Food and Drug Administration (FDA), 57,
139, 146
Forgive and Remember (Bosk), 123
Forrest Gump, 20
Fost, N. C., 201n.36
Frank, Anne, 95
Frank, Arthur, 124, 204n.90
Fredrickson, Donald, 89
Freedman, Benjamin, 142, 205n.105
Freud, A., 202n.48
Freud, Sigmund, 51

Garbarino, J., 200n.23
Gastroenterologists, 25
Geertz, C., 200n.15
Ginzberg, E., 199n.2
Glew, Robert, 66
The Globe, 128
Goldstein, J., 59, 202n.48
Goodman, Ellen, 128
Greene, Graham, 195–196, 206n.127
Gregory, David, 124, 204n.94
Grieco, M. H., 205n.102
Group practices, 7–8, 22–24
Marshfield Clinic, 24–25
Groves, L. K., 205n.108
Growth hormone (GH) for short children,
54–57, 94, 97, 101
Grumbach, M., 201n.34

Hack, M., 148, 149, 205n.106
Harvard Medical School, 160
Healing the Wounds (Hilfiker), 124
Health care reform, 26, 31, 68, 105, 163,
193–197
Clinton's Health Reform Task Force, 16
future of medical care, 193–194
personal experiences and, 16–21
Work Group on Ethics, 16–18
Health care system
bias in treatment, 141–142
delivery of care, 7–8
doctor as team member, 5–7

as economic business, 3, 16, 22–26, 44, 79, 194
evidence-based medicine, 144
free market and, 194–195
hospital admissions, 189–191
measurement and accountability, 27
medical success and, 163–168, 182–184
mythology of progress, 141, 145
opportunity cost of care, 70, 104–107, 194
patient-protection resources, 154
physician-induced demand for services, 102
public health interventions, 154, 173, 182
rationing of health care, 17, 44, 68, 97
roles and responsibilities, 1–2
scientific bureaucratization of medicine, 170–171
societal changes and, 3–4, 23, 97
Health maintenance organization (HMO), 28, 195–197
Hearing impairments, 57
Hellman, D. S., 136–137, 148, 204n.99
Hellman, Samuel, 136–137, 148, 204n.99
Hilfiker, David, 12, 124–125, 199n.5, 204n.93
Hinrz, R. L., 201n.41
Hippocrates, 85, 119, 161–163
Hitler, Adolf, 114
Horbar, J. D., 205n.106
Hospice care, 47
The House of God (Shem), 101
Human Genome Project, 158
Hypertrophic cardiomyopathy (HCM), 99

Iffy, Leslie, 137, 205n.101
Ihongbe, J. C., 202n.54
Indirect myocardial revascularization (IMR), 149
Infant mortality rates, 49, 67, 141
African-American babies and, 103
birthweight-specific mortality rates, 148–149
Informed-consent, 86–89, 112, 151, 153
children and, 90–92
goals of law versus ethics, 90
malpractice cases and, 87
placebo-controlled trials, 134–136

religious beliefs and, 107–111
Ingber, Ellen, 124, 204n.94
Internal medicine, 19, 21
Internet, 83, 91, 98, 122
Iron, T. G., 201n.29
Ishiguro, Kazuo, 131, 204n.98
Israeli, Isaac, 85

Jefferson Medical College, 21
Jewell, S., 202n.50
Johanson, A. J., 201n.41, 202n.44
Johns Hopkins University, 53, 160
Johnson, Lyndon B., 19
Jones, K. L., 200n.21
Jordan, Michael, 102

Kafka, F., 160
Kant, Emmanuel, 50
Kaplan, S. L., 201n.40
Kass, Leon, 98, 161, 162, 163, 203n.75, 205n.112
Kassirer, Jerome, 78, 202n.60
Katz, Jay, 85, 89, 122–123, 203n.64, 204n.86
Kaufman, S. R., 199n.11
Kennedy, John F., 24
Kevorkian, Jack, 94
Kilbourne, Edwin, 137, 205n.101
Kirp, David, 72, 202n.56
Konner, Melvin, 12, 160, 199n.3, 199n.7, 205n.111
Kopelman, A. E., 201n.29
Kopelman, L. M., 201n.29
Kostelny, K., 200n.23
Kramer, Peter, 94, 203n.72
Kukoc, Tony, 102
Kuttner, R., 206n.125
Kuwait, invasion and suffering of children, 49, 64

La Rabida Children's Hospital and Research Center, 37–38
Lantos, Hannah (daughter), 133, 139
Lantos, J. D., 199n.8, 199n.10, 200n.28, 201n.42, 202n.54, 203n.80
Lantos, Jeff (brother), 19
Lantos, Nancy (wife), 11, 29, 93, 96

Lantos, Raymond J. (father), 18–21
  multi-specialty group practice and,
    22–24, 27–28
  personal experiences in becoming a
    physician, 18–21
Lead toxins, 30
*Learning by Heart: AIDS and Schoolchildren
  in America's Communities* (Kirp), 72
Lee, P. D., 201n.38
Lethal injection, 95
Levinson, W., 204n.88, 204n.95
Lewis, Sinclair, 179–181, 191, 206n.123
Lincoln, Abraham, 111
Lipkin, M., Jr., 199n.1
Listening to Prozac (Kramer), 94, 95
Liver disease, 65, 67, 75
Lo, B., 203n.73
Lupus, 34

McCarty, Daniel, 24, 200n.16
McCauthey, E. S., 201n.39
McCormick, R. A., 53, 201n.30
Magaziner, Ira, 17
Maimonides, 161
Mainus, A. G., III, 204n.95
Malaria, 66, 75
Malloy, M. H., 205n.106
Malpractice cases, 87–89, 129; *see also*
  Errors and mistakes
Managed care, 7, 21–22, 27–28, 189
Marshfield Clinic (group practice), 24–25
Measles, 49, 66, 67
Medicaid, 16, 37
Medical College of Wisconsin Bioethics
  Discussion Forum on the Internet,
  83, 203n.63
Medical education, 65, 75–78, 181–182
  as business enterprise, 73–74
  curricular reform, 74, 159–160
  deans' interviews, 160
  errors among trainees, 123
  issues of, 2, 72
  memorization and, 72
  morality and, 65, 68, 76–81
  teacher-student relationship, 78
  teaching rounds, 77
Medical ethics, 14, 48, 53, 67–68; *see also*

Bioethics
  guidelines for research, 88–89, 146, 152
  moral evasion, 119–122
  morality of medicine, 79–81, 112–114
  traditional medical ethics, 86, 161–162
  truth telling and, 82–85
Medical futility, 70–71, 97
  Baby L case, 71–72
Medical progress, 141, 145, 152–156
  medical science and, 148–150
  medical success and, 163–168, 182–184
  regulating progress, 150–152
Medical testing; *see* Clinical drug testing
Medicare, 16, 24, 77
Meningitis, 75
Miles, S. H., 199n.10
Mill, John Stuart, 62, 202n.52, 202n.53
Mnookin, R., 202n.47
Moby Dick (Melville), 28
Monetarization of health care, 3
Moral theory, 62–65, 96, 101, 132
The Moviegoer (Percy), 171, 173
Mulligan, J., 201n.39
Murphy, R. F., 203n.66
Muyskens, J., 201n.33
My Own Country (Verghese), 29

Narrative ethics, 164
Natason v. Kline, 87, 203n.68
National Association for the Deaf (NAD), 57,
  202n.46
National Heart Institute, 89
National Institutes of Health (NIH), 55, 79,
  99, 136
Needleman, Jacob, 79, 170, 206n.119
Neonatal care, 54, 57, 116–118, 131,
  148–149
  patent ductus arteriosus (PDA) clinical
    trials, 134–135
New England Journal of Medicine, 19, 49,
  71, 77, 124, 136
New York Times, 74, 98, 105
New Yorker, 140
Newton, Isaac, 112
Nickerson, K. G., 202n.59
Nigeria, 66–67
Nixon, Richard, 189

Non-heart-beating cadavers, 68
Nutritionists, 7

Objectivity, 164
Obstetrics, 21
Occupational therapists, 7
Oe, Kenzaburo, 40, 42, 200n.24
Omene, J. A., 202n.54
Open Heart (Yehoshua), 175–178
Operation Wandering Soul (Powers), 44, 89,
    172, 178, 192–193
Opportunity costs of care, 70, 104–107, 194
Oral contraceptives, 5
Organ transplants, 5, 69, 73, 79, 100
Orthopedics, 33

Pardo, C., 200n.23
Paris, J. J., 202n.55
Passamani, Eugene, 137, 148, 204n.100
Pasteur, Louis, 74, 137
Patent ductus arteriosus (PDA), 134–135
Patient empowerment, 82
    children as patients, 90–92
Patient-controlled analgesia (PCA), 185–186
Pediatrics, 21, 25, 54
    informed consent and, 90–92
Pellegrino, Edmund, 161–163, 205n.113
Pensack, Robert, 98–102, 124, 203n.77,
    204n.92
Percival, Thomas, 85, 161
Percy, Walker, 78–79, 113, 171, 204n.81,
    206n.120
Peter Pan (Barrie), 44
Pharmacists, 7
Physical therapists, 7
Physician-assisted suicide, 43, 46–47,
    94–95
Pimping (teaching rounds), 77
Pippin, Scottie, 102–103
Placebo-controlled, double-blind testing,
    134–135
    thrombolytic drugs, 138–139
The Plague (Camus), 19, 76–77, 80
Poland, Ron, 137, 205n.101
Postmortem examinations, 129
The Power and the Glory (Greene), 195–196
Powers, Richard, 44–45, 89, 172, 174,

200n.25, 203n.70, 206n.121,
    206n.124
Premature newborns, 15, 45, 52–54, 95,
    116–118; *see also* Neonatal care
Preventive medicine, 80
Proudfit, W. L., 205n.107
Psychiatrists, 58, 102

Quinlan, Karen, 119

Raban, Jonathan, 140, 205n.104
Racism, 103
Radiology, 21
Raising Lazarus (Pensack and Williams), 98
Randomized controlled trials (RCTs),
    136–138, 143, 146–148
    thrombolytic drugs, 138, 150
Rational self-interest, 61
Rationing of health care, 17, 44, 68, 97
Reardon, F., 202n.55
*Recognizable Patterns of Human
    Malformation* (Smith), 32
Reimbursement for services, 2, 37
Remains of the Day (Ishiguro), 131
Renal failure, 34, 38, 45, 55
Respiratory Syncitial Virus infections, 75
Respiratory therapists, 7, 155
Richman, D. D., 205n.102
Ritalin, 94
Rockefeller Institute, 179
Rosenfeld, R. G., 201n.38, 201n.41
Roth, Herman, 120
Roth, Philip, 120, 124, 204n.85, 204n.89
Rothman, D. J., 203n.69
Rubenstein-Taybi syndrome, 116
Rush, Bobby, 190
Russel-Silver syndrome, 116

Sacks, Oliver, 124, 203n.65, 204n.91
Saenger, P., 201n.33
Salgo, Martin, 87
*Salgo v. Leland Stanford University Board of
    Trustees*, 203n.67
Sarfeh, James, 124, 204n.94
Scarification, 43
Schiedermayer, David, 24, 200n.16
Schuit, Ken, 65, 74–75, 78, 80

Sex selection, 68
Shea, Steven, 77, 202n.59
Shem, Samuel, 12, 101, 199n.4
Shields, J. Dunbar, 22–24
Shirey, E. K., 205n.107
Sickle-cell anemia, 34, 185–187, 196
Siegel, P. T., 201n.37
Siegler, M., 201n.42
Silent World of Doctor and Patient (Katz), 85, 122
Silverman, William, 53–54, 201n.32
Silvers, J. B., 201n.43
Silverstein, M., 199n.10
Simon, Paul, 102, 203n.78
Singh, J., 201n.43
Slow code CPR, 43
Smallpox, 4–5
Smith, David, 32–33
Smith-Lemli-Opitz Syndrome, 116
Social workers, 7, 58
Society for Pediatric Research, 92, 103
Solnit, A., 202n.48
Somers, Anne, 22, 200n.12
Somers, H. M., 200n.12
Sones, F. M., Jr., 149, 205n.107
Specialization, 7, 25
    managed care and, 21–22
Spicer, C. M., 162, 205n.114
Stabler, B., 201n.37
Star Trek, 14
Stocking, C. L., 199n.10
Strazl, Thomas, 73
Styne, D. M., 201n.40
Surgery, as specialization, 21, 25, 78

Tenenbaum, J., 202n.59
The Thanatos Syndrome (Percy), 113
Third-party payment, 7
Tolstoy, Leo, 120, 204n.84

Truth telling, 82–86; *see also* Informed consent
    historical context and, 86–90
    Internet forum on, 83–84
    opportunity costs and, 104–107
Tulsky, J., 199n.8
Turner syndrome, 55

University of Benin, Benin City, Nigeria, 66, 75
University of Chicago, 80, 119, 136
University of Pittsburgh School of Medicine, 65, 69, 72–73
USA Today, 69
Uterine cancer, 107

Van Vliet, G., 201n.40
Veatch, R. M., 162, 163, 205n.114
Verghese, Abraham, 12, 29–30, 199n.6, 200n.19
Vinson, D. C., 204n.95
Voss, L. D., 201n.39

Wall Street Journal, 98, 105
The Way of the Physician (Needleman), 79, 170
Weaver, Randy, 190
Wegman, M. E., 203n.79
Western Psychiatric Institute and Clinic, 73
Williams, Dwight, 98, 203n.77, 204n.92
Williams syndrome, 116
Williams, William Carlos, 113–114, 204n.82
Wolf, Susan, 23, 200n.14
Woolf, Virginia, 80
Workman's Compensation, 16

Yehoshua, A. B., 175, 177–178, 206n.122
Young, Quentin, 189

Toulmin, Stephen, 98, 203n.74
Toxicity of treatments, 87
Traven, B., 29, 200n.18